MAGGIE JONES was born in L   worked for the Family Planning Association and the National Council for Voluntary Organisations before becoming a freelance journalist, writing for *The Sunday Times*, *Observer*, *The Guardian* and *The Independent* as well as a variety of women's magazines. She is a breastfeeding counsellor for the National Childbirth Trust and the author of eleven books on health and childcare issues. She is married and has three children.

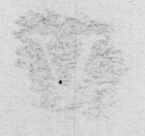

CHOOSING OLDER MOTHERHOOD

The essential guide to becoming a mother over 35

Maggie Jones

Foreword by
Professor Ian Craft FRCS, FRCOG

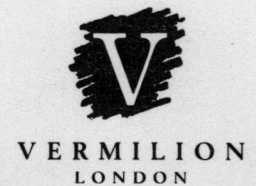

VERMILION
LONDON

First published in the United Kingdom
by Vermilion in 1996

Copyright © Maggie Jones 1996

A CIP catalogue record for this book is available from the
British Library

ISBN 0 09 181302 6

Typeset by M Rules
Printed and bound in Great Britain by
Mackays of Chatham PLC
Chatham, Kent

Vermilion
An imprint of Ebury Press
Randon House
20 Vauxhall Bridge Road
London
SW1V 2SA

Contents

Foreword

How refreshing it is to find a book specifically focused on older-age parenthood. Modern society has become so mesmerised into thinking that those wishing to have a family over the age of 40 are particularly selfish, and that their resultant children will inevitably be disadvantaged in emotional and other ways. Until now, informative and sensible literature on this subject has been lacking.

Our present society has short memories, since natural fertility does normally occur beyond this watershed of age, even allowing for the fact that there is an increased incidence of chromosomal abnormalities and miscarriage. We are now less aware of older-age couples having children simply because many fertile women who would have previously had large families into their late forties, now elect to have a sterilisation procedure, or a termination for an unplanned pregnancy.

However, for those having their first child at this time, whether from natural fertility, or as a result of assisted conception, pregnancy does present an unchartered course full of anxieties and expectations, which appear to be disproportionally exaggerated by the reaction of both the public and even of some members of the medical profession itself.

Maggie Jones's book has much to commend it. It is easily readable and written in a way that most people will understand. Its logical layout starts from the decision-making process about wanting to be pregnant at an age when some of us might expect to be grandparents, and then rightly draws attention to the increased difficulty of becoming parents with conventional, and indeed, assisted conception treatment, including IVF and other related methods. Even so, the author correctly indicates that the availability of egg donation has transformed the prospects of success of fertility treatment, which means that having a family is now more, rather than less, likely for those fortunate enough to be able to receive this method of treatment.

Her descriptive chapters of what to expect when pregnancy does result, of antenatal screening and birth, are liberally interspersed with quotes from real couples expressing both negative and positive reactions, about different experiences, even when they are rightly or wrongly critical of the medical profession. Such responses indicate the author's honest journalism which allows the reader to identify with how they would react in similar circumstances.

In short, this book can be commended to all those who hope to experience one of life's recurring marvels – that of the generation and birth of a new being to a couple who, despite their anxiety about becoming parents at an older age, wish to share the overwhelming joy of becoming a family.

Ian Craft, FRCS, FRCOG

Introduction

More and more women today are choosing to have their babies later in life – that is, in their thirties and early forties. Statistics from the Office of Population Censuses and Surveys show that, yes, late motherhood is definitely on the increase. The average age at which women have their first child is the highest ever at 28 years. Women are now far more likely to have children in their early 30s than their early 20s – a reversal of the situation only five years earlier. In 1993, 87 children were born per 1,000 women aged between 30 and 34, compared with 82 per 1,000 women between 20 and 24. As recently as 1981 the figures were 70 and 107.

Births to women over 40 have risen by half over the past ten years. The statistics also show that an increasing proportion of these births were first births, pointing to a definite trend towards later child bearing. They also show that this tendency to have babies late was most common in middle-class families; nearly half of the births within marriage to the over thirties were to women whose husbands were in professional and managerial occupations.

Between 1980 and 1990 the number of births outside

marriage to women over 30 trebled. It is estimated that about three-quarters of these births were to divorced or separated women. Many of these women were living with their new partners; in 1990, two-thirds of the births outside marriage to older women were registered by both parents living at the same address.

While most women who delay motherhood choose to have children in their late thirties, a few decide to become mothers for the first time in their forties. Recently, many career women have embarked on motherhood very late in their lives, presenting the image of the youthful, sexy, attractive older mother. Actress Patricia Hodge gave birth to her two sons at the ages of 42 and 45. Felicity Kendall also became a first time mother at the age of 41, and in the States, Priscilla Presley gave birth to her son at the age of 42. Many media personalities had their career first and then embarked on motherhood before it was too late – the first of Esther Rantzen's three children was born when she was 38.

Late motherhood is also more common in London and the South-East. Statistics published in the 1993 report Regional Trends showed that in the London area, ten out of every 1,000 births in London in 1991 were to women aged 40 and over, compared with six out of 1,000 in 1981. These figures gave rise to a wave of articles talking about the boom in fertility for the over-forties. In fact, the numbers of births to women in their forties has actually declined in past decades, despite the recent trend in late births. Figures for the year 1938 show that of 621,000 births, 24,474 were to women aged 40–44 and 2,085 to women aged 45–49. In 1951 the proportions were about the same, but by 1971 – after contraception had become widely available and abortion was legalised – the proportion of births to women over

40 had dropped by well over a half, and to women over 45 by two-thirds of the 1951 figure. But most of these late births were the last child in a larger family.

Many pregnancies to older women are still accidental, as is shown by the number of abortions to women over 40 today. In 1991, 9,316 women aged 40–44 had babies, while 5,330 chose to have a termination of pregnancy. During the same year, 519 women aged 45 and over chose to give birth, while 456 chose to have an abortion.

Although the menopause in most women occurs some-time between the age of 45 and 55, most women trying to have a baby in their forties will experience fertility problems. Now new infertility treatment has given hope to older women unable to conceive naturally. The news in 1992 that a British woman aged 58 had conceived twins was greeted with controversy and confusion. Public debate centred on whether it was 'right' for a woman who could be a grandmother to give birth and whether she would be an adequate mother for her children, as well as whether it was moral for doctors to use artificial means to induce a pregnancy in women over the natural age of child rearing. The fact that women as old as 62 have been helped in this way has caused a great deal of public unease.

But what is the 'natural' age at which fertility ends? The oldest mother on record appears to be Mrs Ruth Kistler of Los Angeles who gave birth to her daughter at the age of 57 years, 129 days. In Britain, Kathleen Campbell gave birth in 1987 to her son Jobey at the age of 55. Her baby was conceived naturally – and accidentally – when her youngest child was 16.

The reduction in the numbers of women who have very late babies has probably changed people's attitudes so that it seems more 'unnatural' for women to have a very late baby than it seemed to earlier generations. For women to have a late baby by accident seemed to require help and sympathy, while to choose to have a baby late – perhaps with help from medical science – seems to give rise to judgemental attitudes. Late motherhood is seen as an indulgence in a generation of women who want to 'have it all'; it is not meant to be good for the baby.

Everyone seems to accept that late motherhood carries some risks – for the woman's health, the baby's health, and perhaps their happiness later on. But what are the risks of late motherhood? What chances is the older mother taking with her health and life? What are the chances of her succeeding in having a healthy pregnancy and normal labour? What are the risks of having an abnormal baby? And how successful is parenthood for the older mother, her family, and, especially, for the child? This book will try to answer all of these questions for any of you who are considering having a baby later in life.

1

Making the decision

Women today are able to plan when to have a family as they have never been able to before. The free availability of contraception and legal abortion have meant that, at least in theory, few women feel they have to have a child until they consider they are ready.

Today's women, too, expect to find fulfilment not only through being a wife and mother but also through their careers. The number of women in full-time employment has increased and the introduction of maternity leave legislation in the 1970s means that women can choose to have babies knowing that their job will be held open for their return. More and more women are choosing to postpone having their first child to fit in with their lives, marriages and careers.

Irrational choices

Most of us believe that we make real choices, that children are born out of a rational decision, but interviews with older mothers show that this is very far from the case.

Careless use of contraception, 'feeling broody', a decision suddenly made because a sister or best friend has a baby, boredom or lack of satisfaction with a job, doubts about one's fertility, and fear that 'time is running out' and that the choice may be taken away all seem more common answers to the question, 'What made you decide to have a baby?' than 'We felt it was the right time'. Perhaps such reasons are more common among late mothers; perhaps more women who 'choose' to have their families would decide to have two children, two or three years apart, in their late-twenties or early-thirties.

Most women probably do not 'plan' their families in the accepted sense. Many women feel ambivalence about whether or when to have a child; a wanted pregnancy can finish as a termination, especially when a partner rejects the idea of a baby or the woman's circumstances change – and an unwelcome pregnancy can become a much loved child. All contraceptive methods have a failure rate, especially when used over ten years or so, and women's doubts about their fertility, especially with increasing age, may lead them to 'take risks' to see whether they can conceive. Many women find it takes them longer to conceive than they thought – the average time is 6 months – and others experience problems with their fertility or have miscarriages.

There is very little research on the reasons why women have children late. One study, carried out by Kate Windridge and Judy Berryman at Leicester University, looked at 346 women who had babies at the age of 40 or later. One hundred were first time mothers. They were not representative of the population at large – they responded to advertisements in women's magazines and periodicals, and were mostly in non-manual or professional occupations – but the findings are still very interesting. Only 5 per cent said they had delayed having their babies for career reasons, less than half of the babies were planned, and 40 per cent of the first time mothers over 40 had sought advice on fertility problems, so infertility may have been responsible at least in part for a delay in becoming a mother.

For some women, the decision is an uncomplicated one. 'I had always thought that my mid-thirties was about the right time to have children', says Jenny. 'It gave us five years to enjoy being a couple, having adventurous holidays and that kind of thing, and also earning enough to get the house how we wanted it. I was a bit worried about my fertility declining, so I didn't want to leave it later than 35. In the event it took four months to get pregnant, I took maternity leave, and then I had my second child two years later. I'm still working part time, we have a fantastic nanny, and everything's worked out really well for us.'

For many women, however, reality doesn't work out quite as simply as this. Susie had her first baby at 38 and her second at 42. 'A friend of mine, a GP, got married at 34, decided to start a family two years later at the same time as me, wanted the babies to be born in the spring, and got pregnant straight away, had a boy in April, and two years later, a girl in May. I just can't stand it. It took me nearly two years to get pregnant. Then I had a miscarriage. I had my first child, but then I had another two miscarriages before I had my second child four years later. It was very frustrating. I thought that I could plan everything, but sometimes you just can't. There's so much talk about choice these days; nature has her way sometimes of getting her revenge.'

Even if women feel they do have a choice, however, making that choice is not always easy. Some women postpone having a baby from year to year, looking forward to a perfect time for bringing a child into the world. 'When I have got my promotion . . . when we have moved to a bigger house . . . once we have got some money saved . . .' Postponement can become a way of life, and it is easy to put off the child-bearing decision year after year until suddenly there seems to be no time left.

This is what happened to Tessa, now aged 41. 'At first I was enjoying my job so much that I didn't want to take a break to have a baby. I was working as a journalist and there were lots of exciting opportunities for me; I worked late a lot, and I knew that if I had a child I wouldn't be able to concentrate on my job in the same way.

'Then we decided to move to a bigger house which needed a lot of work doing to it. The work went on for two years and just when we felt we were getting there I got a job in Manchester and we moved again. By now having a child seemed a major upheaval and I didn't want to face it. I saw friends of mine becoming non-people, droning on about nappies and lack of sleep, and I didn't want the same thing to happen to me.

'Now I'm not sure that I shall ever have a child. I'm not using contraception, I haven't for six months, but nothing's happened. Perhaps I've left it too late. But on the other hand, part of me feels relief that I haven't got pregnant. I certainly wouldn't go rushing to the infertility clinic if nothing happened, but if I did get pregnant, then I guess I'd give it a whirl.'

Hilary too had doubts about having a child, although she decided to go ahead before it was 'too late'. 'It was a very conscious decision to have a baby, a decision which I had put off making for many years. I was 38 when we started trying, it took four months to conceive, and I was just 39 when our daughter was born.

'When we married ten years ago we always thought we would have kids. Alan wanted them more than me but he left the decision to me because he knew that I would do the lion's share of everything, and that my life would be most changed. I wasn't very keen – I didn't think the world was a brilliant place to bring someone into, and I didn't think I'd make a wonderful mother. Also my own childhood wasn't happy; I had an older brother who bullied me and I didn't feel I had any support from my parents.

'I think we realised as I got into my late thirties that we were leaving things rather late. I didn't feel that I wanted a baby now, but I thought that if I left it too late I would regret it. I also thought of Alan – it seemed a natural, normal thing to do to have a baby and I didn't want to deprive him of that. People kept telling me having a child was just the greatest thing and I thought I'd probably feel the same if I did it, after all, we're programmed that way.'

Couples who get married young may postpone having children because they feel too immature to cope with the demands that children will make. 'I think we both felt that we needed time together as a couple, to mature, to get to know one another. Then that got to be our state of mind; we wanted to put ourselves and our marriage first, and children were a threat. We kept thinking, will having children spoil our relationship? Will we be driven apart by parenthood?'

Alison recalls that for many years the idea of having a child was too constricting. 'We were both having a good time in our careers, and children would have got in the way. There were times when he wanted a child and I said, "No, not yet", and times when I suggested it and he said, "Maybe next year". We were never sure that we wanted children at the same time until it became necessary to have them because I was getting on. I think I was scared of the responsibility.'

For those who have been married for some time, having a baby later means disrupting a familiar life structure and creating upheaval in a long-established relationship. As they watch their friends and colleagues having children and see the disruption, exhaustion and lack of money it seems harder and harder to make the decision. 'I wanted to have a baby, but quite frankly I was terrified. When I woke up on a Sunday to a leisurely morning reading the papers and then an outing to an art gallery in the afternoon I kept thinking, this wouldn't be possible with kids. I kept thinking, do I really want it? And I really didn't know.'

Some women find the desire for parenthood creeping up on them unawares. Many women described their feelings at this time as 'getting broody'. Kate, 38 when she had her first child, described her broodiness like this: 'I think I found that I was watching other people with babies or young children with great curiosity, thinking, so that's what they do at that age, that woman is breast feeding, or I don't think that was a good way to handle that situation, I would have done it differently. When I really realised what was happening was when I started looking at baby clothes in the local stores and avidly reading magazine articles about natural childbirth.'

For others, it's a realisation that career and home is not enough. 'I'd been working in the agency for 16 years and I'd really done well and enjoyed it, but suddenly I felt I was seeing the same thing over and over. Young people would come in, bursting with ideas, and I'd say, "Oh, we had that 7 years ago, so-and-so did it, try something new." But for them, and for a lot of other people, it *was* new. It was beginning to get repetitious and I felt I was getting stale; I just couldn't summon the enthusiasm I used to have. I wanted something totally different, a new challenge, and that's what motherhood meant.'

Many women find themselves unable to make a positive decision to have children, but may make a more passive one. After all, to prevent pregnancy most women have to take the active step of using contraception. Celia, at 37, made the decision with her partner to come off the pill. 'I felt I'd been taking it long enough and I wanted a change. I was fitted with a cap, and I used that very religiously for about two years. Then I really got bored with it. I felt I'd been messing around with contraception all these years, first with an IUD, then the pill, then the cap. I'd had enough of it. And we'd start getting careless, and taking risks. Then one day I got pregnant. I had no idea how I would react, but in fact I was pleased – I thought, so I really can do it after all. It felt different, somehow very grown up.'

While many women do 'choose' to have a baby later in life, for many circumstances dictate when they have a baby. Harriet had a first child at 39 because she didn't meet her husband until she was 37. 'I had several relationships, but none of them were right. The first man I lived with said he didn't want to have children, ever. With the second man the relationship didn't work out and then I had a long period in which I had a passionate relationship with a man who was hopelessly unreliable; we never lived together and having a child would have been out of the question. When I met

Martin I knew right away this was it. We were both keen to have children and I got pregnant just before we married last year.'

Denise was 41 when she conceived her first child. 'It wasn't as simple as just career reasons, although that was part of it. My first marriage broke up partly as a result of my career – I was more successful than he was. My career took me abroad as a foreign correspondent . . . For some years I wasn't in a relationship where I could have a child. Then I remarried in 1991 and we both wanted children.'

'Not finding the right person' is a common cause of delayed parenthood. Some women go through the agonising process of wondering whether to get pregnant anyway and become a single mother by choice. 'When year after year went by and I didn't get married, I did seriously think about having a baby on my own,' says Debbie, now 40. 'It was very tempting but I kept thinking is it fair on the child?' When I met Stephen I remember thinking perhaps I should just be careless with contraception and see what happens. In the event he said he would like to have a baby with me before I did.'

Disagreements between couples over when to have a baby can be deeply divisive. Often the woman postpones parenthood for some years until her partner feels ready; sometimes he never does. This happened to Ginny. 'He said at the outset that he didn't really want to have children and I accepted that to begin with. Then I thought that as time went by he would probably change his mind, but he didn't. It's a pity I made such an issue out of it and talked about it so much; it meant I couldn't get pregnant by accident, it would be obvious it was a conscious decision. He was always very careful about contraception and I couldn't have fooled him.

'When I hit 40 things suddenly changed. I found I was hating him, and hating myself for having let him make the decision for me. I should have said, "Having a baby is too important for me. If you won't agree, then I'll leave you." Perhaps if I had issued an ultimatum he'd have changed his mind. I think that if we had actually had a baby, he would have seen it differently and been a good father. I've seen other men not keen on having a baby turn into soppy, doting fathers when the child actually arrives. Now its too late. I cry all the time because I realise I'll never be a mother. It's driving us apart; in the end I may end up with neither husband nor child.'

When the woman postpones child-bearing for her partner the consequences can be even more painful. Ellen went along with her partner's wishes not to have a child; she was enjoying her job and thought he would probably come round. 'But then I felt the biological clock ticking away and I thought, it's now or never. I told him I wanted to have a child and he said he didn't feel ready. I said, "Then it will be too late for me".

'My fortieth birthday came and went and then the bombshell was dropped. He said that he had had an affair with his secretary and that he had made her pregnant. Her family were Catholics and they were going to make her have the baby. He said that he had agreed to pay maintenance for the child but that the affair was over and he didn't want to see the mother again. He told me he was deeply ashamed.

'I forgave him and we stayed together. But he does keep in touch with the mother and he does visit his little daughter. Can you imagine what it makes me feel? The other day we were in the high street and I saw him looking at some little girls' shoes in the window of a shop and wondering whether to get them for her. Pain went through me like a knife; I think of that little girl all the time, it torments me, especially at night. He says now that he'd be prepared for me to have a child but I'm 42 and nothing is happening. I should have trusted my instincts and not listened to him.'

Some women go ahead and have a baby despite their partner's opposition, either by an accidental pregnancy or by 'tricking him into it'. Sometimes all works out well; other times it doesn't. Greg expressed his resistance to having children over many years until his wife became pregnant through a genuine accident. 'I had used the cap for over ten years and I guess over that time the chances of something going wrong must be pretty high.' The couple discussed having an abortion and Greg agreed that if she didn't want to have one it would be cruel for him to insist on it. She had the baby but throughout the pregnancy he remained cool and uninvolved. After the baby was born Greg retreated more and more into his job, until he finally left her altogether.

For all those who have delayed parenthood must come some ultimate moment of truth, a realisation that they have not made the decision to have a child and will therefore remain childless. Zoë Wanamaker plays 40-something Tessa Piggott who has a late baby in the TV series *Love Hurts*. Wanamaker herself is 43 and says the timing has never been quite right for her to have a baby, although she says she has not ruled out the possibility altogether. 'You have to be a realist and not a romantic about children. It's easy to fantasise about having a baby . . . I'm not sure it's right for me at the moment.'

The woman who at 43 has still not decided to have a baby will probably join the increasing numbers of women who are choosing never to have children. Recent statistics have shown a definite increase in the number of women choosing to remain childless. Of women born in 1945, 12 per cent were childless at the age of 35, compared with 20 per cent for women born 10 years later. Although there is a shift towards later child-bearing, statistics show that this increase in childlessness is likely to continue among younger women.

Apart from those who decide not to have children, there are those who very much want children and are unable to have them. In fact, with the tremendous advances that have been made in infertility treatment over the past two decades, the number of infertile couples who will never succeed in having a baby may be very small. A study carried out by Gina Johnson among general practice records in South Bedfordshire showed that of 474 women born in 1950, 24 had consulted a doctor about infertility but only five were childless due to unresolved infertility. However, 34 of them were voluntarily childless.

For those who have, for whatever reason, postponed having a baby into their mid to late thirties, infertility can be a devastating blow. 'I know we've read about it in the papers and I knew it was a risk, but I still didn't think it would ever happen to me,' says Gina, 37. 'After six months of trying I went to the GP and he said, "Give it time, you're not as fertile as you were. If you haven't conceived in another six months we'll do something". I hadn't, so back to the GP. We were referred to a clinic, but it was three months ahead. Still nothing happened. We started investigations. These went on for months; each test seemed to be done only at the most fertile time of the month, so that took months to arrange. In the end they discovered I had blocked tubes, probably as a result of an appendicitis operation I had when I was a teenager. The discovery that there really was something wrong was terrible, appalling. And I felt I only had about three years left.'

Gina conceived two years later on her second attempt at IVF (*in vitro* fertilisation).

Many women feel that infertility is a terrible irony after years of using contraception. 'I was on the pill for twelve years. Then I discovered that I was never ovulating to begin with. Those pregnancy scares I had when I'd taken chances before I went on the pill, all those years of swallowing hormones – it all seemed so pointless. I was really angry and distressed.'

Rachel had always wanted children, but didn't marry until she was 36. 'We tried for a baby straight away. Nothing happened. After about nine months we started to do temperature charts. They seemed to show I was ovulating, and so then there was this awful business of trying to time sex for the most fertile time in my cycle. These temperature charts started to dominate our sex life – Paul said he couldn't bear to be told to perform to order, that I was being neurotic. Once he found it wasn't his sperm which were at fault he lost interest in the whole investigation. I felt completely devastated – if I didn't have children what else was there to look forward to? The menopause, old age, death?'

Those who remain childless, whether by choice or not, often find themselves put under considerable pressure by others. Questions such as, 'Well, when are you going to have a baby then?' or 'Don't you think it's selfish not to have children?' are frequently asked. Some women do feel pressured into having a child by the outside world. 'I had been putting it off and putting it off, and I'm not sure that I really wanted a child, but then I thought, this is something almost everybody does. Am I going to feel I've been missing out?' Pressure is put on women to have children by family and friends anxious that the mother shouldn't regret her decision; and notoriously by parents wanting to have grandchildren.

'My mother went on and on about having a grandchild and finally I said, "My career is important to me. If I have a baby will you mind it while I go back to work?" She agreed and it has worked out really well for us.' Others are not so lucky or do not give in to parental pressures; this can cause a lot of stress in family relationships. 'My mother went on about it so much, how unhappy I was making her, that she couldn't see the point in life if she didn't have grandchildren, that I started really avoiding her. Not only does she not have a grandchild, she'll lose her daughter too.'

But, again, the choice to remain childless sometimes comes unstuck with a late and unexpected pregnancy. Then the woman has to make an often painful choice; to have a baby or an abortion. 'I was 40, we'd been married three years and agreed that children weren't on the cards. When I got pregnant it was a terrible shock to me. My partner said, "Well, why don't you just have the baby? It might be nice, after all, to have a kid." I said, "But it's all right for you, you don't have to go through pregnancy, birth, everything. If you change your mind you can walk out." All the same, it didn't seem right at all to have an abortion. I kept thinking, this may be the only chance I ever have to have a baby. Supposing I had an abortion and then changed my mind? I'd never be able to live with myself if I thought I'd thrown away my one chance.'

'Getting pregnant made me realise how ambivalent my feelings were about this whole motherhood thing,' recalls

Gail, who had her first and only baby at 41. 'I'd been quite happy not to have a child and when I thought I might be pregnant I felt really awful, worried, confused. But then when I got the result of the pregnancy test I felt over the moon. I think I have never felt so happy; I was so excited and I felt, I know it sounds awful, I felt so womanly, somehow.'

For the woman who is much older, pregnancy can seem too remote to be something that can be counted on. 'When I remarried in my early forties I thought we wouldn't have a child,' says Ann, who had three children from her former marriage, then almost grown up. 'I did think that it would be a pity if John, who was 12 years younger than me, couldn't have had a child because of my age. I had a miscarriage when I was 44 and that was sad, a disappointment, because I thought it would be my last chance, but it wasn't a great trauma for me.

'I went back to teaching. I didn't take any precautions and I didn't conceive. Then, two years later, my period was late and I felt terrible. When the pregnancy test proved positive I was very thrilled, but I'd had two miscarriages and I didn't want to get too excited.' A healthy son was born when she was 47.

Heather, who remarried in her mid-thirties, also had miscarriages. 'I thought it was too late and that I probably wouldn't succeed in having a baby. I thought it was all too much trouble and I wasn't sure I wanted to try again. The doctors said I should wait before trying again in any case, so I asked Stephen to use a sheath. He was rather careless about it and I conceived, so Margaret is an accident after three miscarriages!'

The much older mother may not even be aware that she has conceived. Marilyn was 43 with two grown-up sons when her periods became rather irregular. 'I put down the lack of periods to my age, and since I'd always gained weight very easily, I didn't really notice what was happening. When I finally went to the doctor and had a pregnancy test I discovered that I was already 20 weeks pregnant, really too late to have an abortion.'

Accidental pregnancies later in life can cause women – and their partners – a great deal of heart-searching. 'I was 45 when I discovered I was pregnant – I'd become a bit careless about contraception, I really didn't think I was fertile any more. At first I thought I'd have a termination, and told my GP so, but one night I just said, "Suppose I have the baby?" and we talked about it and then decided to go ahead. We both loved one another, we felt we could cope with a baby, and I still feel deep down that taking life is wrong. At the same time, I feel I could easily have had an abortion, and I have great sympathy with any woman who finds herself having to make the difficult choice. And if Len had said no it would have been very different, there's no way I would have had the baby without his support.'

Second time around

Another reason for the increase in births to older mothers is the increasing incidence of divorce and remarriage. Many women who have completed their first family, split up, remarry or live with a new partner and want to have a child to seal the relationship. This can be especially important when the new partner has not had children before.

'When I married Steve I had two teenage children and he

had a daughter, aged four, from his previous marriage. We both very much wanted to have another baby although I was nearly 40. It seemed to us that having another baby would bring the whole family together, and it also seemed a good idea to provide a brother or sister for Laura, who wanted this very much.'

Ann was 47 when she gave birth to her fourth child; her other three children from her first marriage were in their early twenties. 'John was 14 years younger than me and although we'd discussed children and decided it was fine not to have them, I did feel that it would have been a pity if my age would have prevented him being a father. He was good with children – everyone's wonderful uncle and godfather. In the event its been absolutely the right thing, it's been wonderful for him to have a child.'

Earth mothers

Another group of older mothers are those who have large families, sometimes spreading over many years. These are the 'earth mothers' who find having a small baby at the breast the most fulfilling time of their lives and are reluctant to move on. Sally married at 32 and had four children when she was 33, 35, 37 and 39. Then, unable to leave the experience behind her, she had another 'last minute' fifth child at the age of 43.

'I'm quite prepared to admit that there might be something wrong with me, that I had all these children for my own pleasure and that I'm postponing facing up to life beyond small children, but they're all healthy, they're all happy, I believe you get to be a much better mother with experience, so I don't think anyone should really criticize me. And if anyone mentions the population problem, I just say my sister doesn't want children so she's let me have her 2.3 for her.'

Afterthoughts

Other late babies are born to women much later, after the mother has decided that her family is complete. Most of these late babies are 'mistakes', or 'afterthoughts', but some are planned. James and Fiona had been married for 15 years and had two teenage children when Fiona found that James had been having an affair. 'This really shook things up, and for some weeks things were fairly desperate,' recalls Fiona. But the couple had a strong relationship, and found that the affair brought up hidden dissatisfactions which, once aired, helped bring them closer together again. 'We went away and had a second honeymoon. I suggested another baby, and to my amazement James agreed with me, and Marianne was the result. She has been wonderful, an absolute joy to the whole family, she's brought us all closer together, including the children.'

Single women

A woman living on her own reaching her late thirties may decide she cannot wait any longer to find the 'right man' or may not even want to live with a man, but may still want a child. More women than ever are deciding to go it alone, partly because social attitudes to single mothers have changed and become more accepting. Women may either choose to conceive through a male friend, either with his consent or by stealth, or may seek artificial insemination by donor. Not all doctors will provide this opportunity to single women, and especially to lesbian women, but there are doctors who are willing.

For all older women who decide to get pregnant, however, there are two main worries; will I conceive, and how long will it take me – and will I be able to have a normal pregnancy and birth, and a healthy child?

2

If you can't get pregnant

Infertility and late motherhood are linked in two ways – first, many women come late to motherhood because they have had trouble conceiving, and second, fertility declines with age and many women who leave it to their mid- or late-thirties or early-forties to have a child will often experience some difficulty in getting pregnant.

Although every doctor and medical textbook will state that fertility declines with age, finding out exactly when and how fast fertility declines is not so easy. Figures from the Office of Population Censuses and Surveys show that in 1993 9,986 women aged 40–44, and 539 women aged 45 and over gave birth, out of a total of 673,000 births for women of all ages – clearly a minority. This figure doesn't really prove anything, however; the smallness of the figure may be more due to women choosing to have their babies earlier rather than experiencing difficulty in having them later.

A study by Professor Trussel of Princeton University and Dr Wilson of the London School of Economics, which was published in 1985, shows that between the years 1550 and 1849, when people did not have access to birth control, only about 7 per cent of women who married young were infertile, while one-third of women who married at the age of 35 did not give birth and nearly 60 per cent of women who married at 40 had no children.

One recent study to try to answer this question was carried out in the Netherlands on a group of 751 women attending clinics for artificial insemination by donated sperm. This study showed that the decline in fertility began at the age of 31, and that after this age the chance of conceiving per monthly cycle fell by about 12 per cent with each year of age. The chance of a woman aged 35 getting pregnant and giving birth to a healthy baby was about half that of a woman aged 25. The study also showed that for older women, continuing beyond 12 cycles was important, since older women took longer to conceive. While only 54 per cent of women over 31 became pregnant after 12 cycles, 75 per cent did after 24. While these figures may be slightly different to those found from women who conceive normally – it is known that there is a slightly lower rate of conception through donor insemination than natural conception – they are likely not to be too far out.

The reasons for infertility in older women are on the whole the same as those for younger women, except that these problems arise more frequently. Most common is probably a failure to ovulate. As women age, they are likely to have more menstrual cycles without ovulating than younger women; eventually most cycles will be anovulatory, as women usually continue to have periods long after they cease to be fertile, perhaps for some ten years before they reach the menopause.

Older women are also more likely to have suffered from some infection or illness which might cause scarring of the

Fallopian tubes, the second most common cause of female infertility, or to develop fibroids or other disorders of the womb which affect fertility.

Research into infertility and a host of new treatments have meant that more women with fertility problems are able to have a baby than ever before. Advances such as IVF (*in vitro* fertilisation, the 'test tube baby' treatment) have put infertility very much in the public domain, and infertility is no longer the hush-hush issue it used to be. Because of this, many women are now aware that their fertility may be a problem, and are much more likely to seek help quickly if they do not become pregnant soon after stopping contraception.

Women who have spent years on the pill or worrying about contraception, who may never have had an act of unprotected intercourse or fretted till their period turned up if they did, may be surprised to find that pregnancy does not automatically result as soon as they abandon contraception. In fact, it has been estimated that the average length of time for a fertile couple having regular sexual intercourse to conceive a baby is about six months. This means that for every lucky couple who get pregnant the first month, another couple will wait a year. It's rather like trying to throw a 'six' in a game like Ludo – the chance of conceiving each month is probably the same, but for the woman in her late thirties, not conceiving straight away will probably ring alarm bells, and she will be aware all the time that a delay of a year in conceiving may considerably reduce her chances. She may rush off for fertility investigations before she has given her body a chance to conceive naturally.

If a couple have not conceived after a year, and especially if the mother is older, most GPs will be sympathetic in

referring a couple to a fertility specialist to begin investigations into whether there is a problem and what this might
be.

How conception occurs

Human conception is a miraculous and complex event,
and what is surprising is perhaps that pregnancy occurs so
often, rather than that it sometimes fails. A human egg is
released every month from a woman's ovary under the
influence of a complex cycle of hormones released by the
pituitary gland and the hypothalamus. The egg is swept
into the Fallopian tubes by the delicate projections (the
fimbriae) at the end of the tubes, where it is normally fertilised by the man's sperm. The fertilised egg then moves
down the tube and, aided by the tiny hair-like cilia which
line the tube, enters the womb. The embryo must implant
into the lining of the womb (the endometrium) where it
starts to produce hormones which will stimulate its
growth. The body in the ovary, the corpus luteum, from
which the egg was released must produce enough of the
hormone progesterone to sustain the pregnancy until, after
the first three months, the placenta takes over. The
woman's womb must be structurally sound and capable of
expanding to contain the growing foetus and the cervix
strong enough to hold the baby in until it is ready to be
born.

It is estimated that it takes a fertile couple having regular
sexual intercourse an average of six months to conceive. At
any stage, something can go wrong and a pregnancy will
not result:

- Sometimes an egg will not be released.
- The egg and sperm may fail to meet and fertilise.
- Many early embryos fail to implant and sometimes an implanted embryo fails to develop or is rejected by the mother's body.
- An abnormality in the foetus or a lack of sufficient levels of the hormone progesterone may make it impossible for the embryo to survive, resulting in a miscarriage.

Roughly 30 per cent of infertility is caused by a problem in the woman; 30 per cent in the man; 30 per cent by both and about 10 per cent is unexplained. These statistics are repeated in almost every guide to the subject, yet in reality, the figures may be somewhat different. A survey at the Bristol Maternity Hospital showed the main causes of infertility to be ovulatory failure (21 per cent), tubal damage (14 per cent), and sperm defects (24 per cent); 28 per cent had unexplained infertility. The statistics for unexplained infertility have tended to fall with better diagnosis and an improved understanding of what causes infertility, but it is still more common than many doctors like to admit.

The most common cause of female infertility is failure to ovulate, then, and this is the easiest to treat. A course of fertility drugs can be given to see if these will activate the ovaries. There are several fertility drugs, and while the doctor may know which is the best to try, often he simply has to go through each in turn, trying different doses, to see what is or is not successful. This can have the effect of making the woman feel like a human guinea-pig. Tests into other areas of infertility can be long, complicated and invasive. Male infertility is the hardest to treat.

Visiting a fertility clinic

If you eventually visit a fertility clinic, both you and your partner will be asked for details of your medical history: any past illnesses and any surgery. You will also be asked questions about your sex life; how many sexual partners you have had, how often you make love, and so on. Many people find this an intrusion into their privacy, but it is all very relevant.

A routine physical examination will then be carried out on both partners. You will be examined to check that your respective reproductive organs are normal. For the man, this means inspecting the external genitalia and in particular the testicles for any signs of a varicocele or other abnormality. The woman will have an internal pelvic examination, during which the doctor will insert a speculum to hold the walls of the vagina apart so that he can view the cervix and take swabs for testing if he suspects a vaginal infection. He will also use his hands to feel the internal organs; this may enable him to detect problems such as fibroids, ovarian cysts or scarring from previous infections.

Tests undergone by the woman

One of the first tests for infertility is to find out whether the woman is ovulating, by using basal body temperature charts. At the time of ovulation there is a small but distinct rise in the body's temperature, due to production of the hormone progesterone. This can be measured by taking a woman's temperature every morning on waking up, a procedure which many find irksome. A three-monthly record should show if you are ovulating and if your cycle is normal, though you may be asked to continue keeping a temperature chart for much longer than this. Because temperature charts are sometimes difficult to interpret and are not always reliable, the woman will probably be given further tests to measure the level of hormones which control ovulation. A blood progesterone test, which is a simple and painless way of measuring the level of progesterone when it reaches its peak at about day 24 in a 28-day cycle, can be done. If the level of progesterone is high, it is a good indication that ovulation has occurred.

The post-coital test may also pinpoint why a woman is not conceiving. The woman makes an appointment for the time of the month when she thinks she will be ovulating. The couple are asked to have sexual intercourse on the night before or the morning of the appointment. At the clinic, the doctor will take a sample of the woman's cervical mucus from the neck of the womb, for examination. The quality of the mucus – clear and slippery, or sticky and opaque – will tend to indicate whether the woman has ovulated. By examining the mucus under a microscope, it is also possible to tell if the sperm are normal, if there are enough of them and whether the sperm are agglutinated which might indicate the presence of antibodies. If post-coital tests are repeatedly not very good, the next step may be to test the semen and mucus for antibodies to sperm which may interfere with sperm motility.

An endometrial biopsy is a procedure which will show whether or not the woman has ovulated. It involves taking a small sample of the lining of the womb for examination. This is a minor surgical procedure, similar to a D and C. The test should show if the womb lining is sufficiently primed by hormones to be able to receive the egg for implantation. If the woman is ovulating normally, the next line of investigation will be to see if the Fallopian tubes are clear.

A hysterosalpingram is an X-ray of the uterus and Fallopian tubes. A dye is injected through the cervix and into the uterus. The dye passes through the womb, along the Fallopian tubes and into the pelvic cavity, enabling all the organs to be viewed.

A laparoscopy is used to detect blocked or damaged tubes and other abnormalities of the womb or ovaries. Under general anaesthetic, a small incision is made in the navel and a laparoscope – a telescope-like instrument – is inserted, which allows the surgeon to examine the organs in detail and assess the extent of any damage.

Sometimes a hysteroscopy is performed – an inspection of the inside of the womb with an instrument similar to a laparoscope. Ultrasound may also be used vaginally to assess the ovaries and womb.

Tests undergone by the man

The man will be asked to produce one or more sperm samples, and this should be done at the outset, before the woman undergoes any major procedures. The man is asked to produce a sample by masturbation into a sterile container either in the clinic, or at home. If he does this at home, he must deliver the sample to the clinic within one-and-a-half hours. The sample is examined to see if the sperm are healthy, numerous and motile. Since one test is not always reliable, a poor result may mean he has to repeat the test. Sometimes a man is diagnosed as sub-fertile on the basis of one test alone. Yet a single sperm count is very unreliable as an indicator of a man's normal fertility. Sperm counts vary enormously from one act of intercourse to another. If all is well, this may be the only test the man has to undergo. If he has a very low or absent sperm count, however, investigations may be undertaken to see if a cause can be found. The sperm may also be examined by the post-coital test, which may give some insight into why the sperm are not functioning properly.

Hormone tests may also be carried out to check levels of testosterone, a male hormone, and a testicular biopsy may be performed. In some cases where the man has no sperm at all, or azoospermia, an operation may be carried out under general anaesthetic to check that the vas deferens are not obstructed and see whether there are any abnormalities.

Aftermath of contraception

Contraceptive methods are a cause of infertility only very rarely. The inter-uterine device (IUD) can increase a woman's chance of suffering from pelvic inflammatory disease, which can lead to infertility. The contraceptive pill sometimes leads to a condition called post-pill amenorrhoea, in which a woman's periods do not return when she stops taking the pill. Research has shown that this only lasts for a maximum of two years after pill use, and it can also be treated with drugs.

A woman used to taking the pill for several years, or using an IUD or cap regularly and worrying every time her period is late, may well expect to get pregnant as soon as she stops using her chosen contraception – but often does not. This does not necessarily mean that she is infertile. However, as a woman gets older her fertility declines, and using contraception for years may mean she is less fertile when she stops and tries to get pregnant. Also, using contraception, and particularly the pill, can disguise infertility problems for years; the pill usually means that a woman has a regular cycle and so may not realise she is not in fact ovulating.

Hormonal problems

One of the most common causes of infertility in women is a malfunctioning of the complex hormonal interactions which govern a woman's menstrual cycle. The woman's monthly cycle is controlled by the pituitary gland in the brain which, in turn, is governed by another gland called the hypothalamus. The pituitary produces a follicle-stimulating hormone (FSH), which controls the production of the hormone oestrogen by the ovary. It also prepares one of the follicles inside the ovary to release the egg. A second pituitary hormone, luteinising hormone (LH), enables the ovary to release its egg. Oestrogen causes the lining of the womb to thicken in readiness to receive the fertilised egg.

If the egg is not fertilised, the corpus luteum begins to shrink, levels of oestrogen and progesterone decrease, the lining of the womb disintegrates and menstrual bleeding results. The falling levels of oestrogen and progesterone stimulate the pituitary to produce more FSH, and the cycle begins again.

If the egg is fertilised, however, and implants into the womb, the corpus luteum continues to produce oestrogen and progesterone until the placenta attaching the foetus to the wall of the womb is mature enough to produce the necessary hormones itself.

Failure to ovulate is normally caused by the woman's body failing to produce enough of the pituitary hormones, or releasing them at the wrong time. Since the pituitary is ultimately controlled by the hypothalamus, anything which affects the hypothalamus can also affect this gland. The hypothalamus can be affected by severe physical and emotional stress, as many women will know when the stress of travel, work, illness or emotional turmoil disrupts their menstrual cycle. As women age, fewer menstrual cycles actually involve ovulation, so that in her early forties as few as one in every two or three cycles will produce an egg.

Treatment

Help for women unable to ovulate has been available for many years in the form of fertility drugs. There are two main types: those which prod the pituitary into producing FSH and LH on time and those which replace FSH and LH if this approach fails.

Clomiphene (Clomid) is an artificial drug which triggers the release of FSH and LH in the pituitary. It seems to induce ovulation in about 80 per cent of women treated, though not all these will succeed in getting pregnant. One reason for this is that clomiphene tends to prevent the cervical mucus from becoming fluid at the fertile time in the month to enable the sperm to enter the womb. This problem can sometimes be overcome by giving oestrogen as well in the few days before ovulation.

Sometimes a combination of clomiphene and human chorionic gonadotrophin (HCG, a hormone produced by the placenta and young embryo) given on the fourteenth day of the cycle will induce women to ovulate who would not do so on clomiphene alone. Clomiphene also seems to help women with a progesterone deficiency. It has been in use for many years and is considered safe, although a few women do have unpleasant side-effects, such as nausea, feeling bloated, or very rarely, enlargement of the ovaries accompanied by pain in the pelvis. Some infertility specialists deny the severity of these symptoms, or fail to inform women of them. Severe symptoms may indicate over-stimulation of the ovaries.

Recently there has been some concern that clomiphene might cause an increase in the number of eggs released following its use, which have chromosomal abnormalities. Others have questioned whether there might be other long-term effects on the children who are conceived after their mothers took fertility drugs, as happened with women who took the drug DES (diethylstilboestrel) in early pregnancy to prevent a miscarriage. This is of particular concern to women who take large doses of fertility drugs to make them produce more than one egg, or super ovulate, as is done for IVF and other treatments. However, there is no evidence to support such fears as yet.

Human menopausal gonadotrophin (HMG), Pergonal or Humagon, is a hormone extracted from the urine of pregnant women and stimulates the follicles which contain the egg. It is usually given as a daily injection followed by the injection of another drug, HCG, which actually triggers ovulation. About 90 per cent of women will ovulate with this treatment, though again not all will conceive and some will miscarry. About 20–30 per cent of pregnancies resulting from this treatment will be multiple births; HMG is responsible for most of the multiple pregnancies which occur with fertility drugs.

The hormone HMG is very potent and may also over-stimulate the ovaries, so the level of oestrogen in the blood needs to be monitored daily and the follicles are often monitored by ultrasound. A new development which might overcome this problem is a small 'pump' about the size of a pocket book which, attached to the woman's arm, provides small, even doses of hormone through a fine needle.

However, having a pump attached day and night and having to go and have the needle repositioned when necessary can be unpleasant.

Some women do not ovulate because they have in their blood a high level of a hormone called prolactin, which is normally only produced in quantity while breast feeding and tends to prevent ovulation. For women with this problem there may be hope with a drug called bromocriptine. Bromocriptine prevents the pituitary from producing prolactin, and after treatment with it ovulation occurs in about 95 per cent of women who previously produced too much.

Scarring or structural abnormalities

The other major causes of infertility in women are scarring of the reproductive organs by past disease or surgery, or structural abnormalities present from birth.

- Untreated sexually transmitted diseases, especially gonorrhoea, can result in infertility. As many as 80 per cent of infected women never have any severe symptoms with the disease, and may not realise that they have it and infection has spread to the Fallopian tubes, causing damage.
- PID (pelvic inflammatory disease) which can start after an induced abortion or miscarriage, after childbirth, after surgery in the pelvic region or after infection with a sexually transmitted disease, can cause tubal scarring and blockage.
- Other infections which can affect fertility are chlamydia and mycoplasmas. Chlamydia, a bacterium

which closely resembles a large virus, has deceptively mild symptoms and an untreated 'silent' infection can destroy the inside of a woman's Fallopian tubes in a matter of days. Mycoplasmas, another organism, may affect fertility and has been held responsible for miscarriages.

Other causes

Endometriosis is a disease which may affect as many as five to ten per cent of women at some stage in their reproductive lives. The condition is caused by patches of the endometrial tissue which lines the womb, or endometrium, becoming deposited outside the womb. This tissue, like the womb lining, thickens and bleeds with each menstrual cycle. Scar tissue is then formed which may block the ends of the Fallopian tubes, or adhesions may form which prevent the tube from picking up the egg on its release from the ovary.

Endometriosis can be treated by a number of drugs; birth control pills or progesterone, or a drug called Danazol, which blocks production of the two pituitary hormones and now new drugs called LHRH analogs which are given as a nasal spray or injection. The idea is that these treatments 'switch off' the menstrual cycle, stopping the patches of endometrial tissue from bleeding; they will then fade away, and any adhesions or scar tissue can be removed by careful surgery.

About one-third of all women have fibroids or polyps by the age of 40. These are benign swellings in the womb, usually only the size of a grape but sometimes swelling to the size of a grapefruit. Fibroids seldom cause symptoms in women who are not pregnant and rarely cause problems in pregnancy, but women with fibroids may find their fertility is affected. They can be removed by surgery.

Malformations of the womb, such as the presence of a dividing wall or septum, again can sometimes be corrected by surgery.

A further cause of damage to the tubes is previous surgery in the abdominal region. Bleeding or trauma to the tissues may result in the formation of scar tissue or adhesions which may then block or fix the tubes, ovaries or womb into unnatural positions that make it impossible for the egg to pass from the ovaries into the Fallopian tubes, therefore making conception impossible. One leading British micro surgeon who has specialised in repairing damaged Fallopian tubes has criticised surgeons for not taking enough care when operating in the abdominal region of women of childbearing age. Of 108 women with tubal damage referred to the Hammersmith Hospital, London over a three-month period, 73 per cent had had previous pelvic surgery.

Increasing skill in carrying out delicate microsurgery has given more women with blocked Fallopian tubes a chance to achieve pregnancy. However, if surgery is not effective, there is still hope through the test-tube baby treatment or IVF (see Chapter 4).

Occasionally a fertilised egg fails to move down through the tube and into the womb and, instead, grows in the tube. Eventually it will abort, or may burst the tube, causing considerable bleeding and damage. An ectopic or tubal pregnancy thus results in both the loss of one pregnancy and a possible barrier to future conception. One tube is often lost and the other may be damaged by bleeding caused by the tube rupturing, or surgery to remove the pregnancy. It is estimated that about 50 per cent of women who have an ectopic pregnancy may never conceive again, although careful surgery by laparoscopy may increasingly be able to save a tube.

Often an ectopic pregnancy occurs when there has been some damage to the tube, perhaps caused by past infections or surgery. It is also more common if a woman becomes pregnant with an IUD in place or has been using the progestogen only (or 'mini') pill. An ectopic pregnancy is very painful and can be life-threatening. However, prompt medical attention to remove the developing embryo before the tube can burst avoids many risks as well as improving the chances of successfully reconstructing the damaged tube.

Causes of male infertility

Men's fertility also falls with age, though more slowly and later than in women. Since most older mothers have partners the same age or older, male infertility can be involved. A combination of slightly lowered fertility in both partners can combine to make pregnancy less likely.

Male infertility can be caused by blocked tubes, the vasa deferentia, which carry sperm from the testes where they are made to the penis. Tubes can be blocked from birth due to a congenital defect, through scarring caused by sexually transmitted diseases, and through surgery, as in a vasectomy. An increasing number of men choose vasectomy once their families are complete, but if the marriage breaks up and they remarry, vasectomy can be the cause of infertility in the second marriage.

Male infertility can also be caused by:

- undescended testicles – if these are not diagnosed early in a boy's life permanent infertility will result;
- infections involving the testicles – orchitis, inflammation of the testicles following mumps, very occasionally can result in infertility;
- varicocele – a sort of varicose vein of the testicle – which may be a cause of male infertility;
- disorders of ejaculation – sometimes, as a result of illness such as diabetes or surgery such as a prostatectomy, sperm is ejaculated backwards into the bladder at orgasm;
- low sperm count, or a large proportion of the man's sperm being abnormal. Although research is being done, no-one really understands the causes of low sperm counts; however, their origin is believed to be hormonal.

Treatments

Because so little is understood about the causes of much male infertility, very limited help is available for the majority of men with a low or absent sperm count. Some causes are known (see above) but there is little to be done about them.

One form of male infertility can be caused by a varicocele, or varicose vein, around the testicle. This can be treated, although its link with infertility has been questioned. A simple operation to tie off the vein may result in an improvement to sperm quantity and quality in about two-thirds of cases, thus increasing the chances of conception.

Blocked or scarred vasa deferentia, especially after vasectomy, may be restored surgically but there is only a

50 per cent success rate; this is because a man with blocked tubes often produces antibodies to the sperm as they cannot be ejaculated and have to be reabsorbed by the body. Percutaneous epididymal sperm aspiration can now remove sperm from the testes, and be used to fertilise an egg.

Other causes of a low sperm count are very resistant to treatment. Various hormone treatments have been tried, but with a very low success rate. Some studies have shown that the success rate is actually lower among treated men than among those who have not received any drugs at all. Many of the drugs – some of which are the same as female fertility drugs – also have unpleasant side-effects such as loss of libido, swollen breasts or loss of body hair. To a man whose self-esteem is already dented by the fact of his infertility, these side-effects can be impossible to bear and such treatments are seldom used today.

One new technique that may help men with a low sperm count is the split ejaculate technique, where the first part of several ejaculates – the part richest in sperm – is pooled and introduced into the vagina through artificial insemination. This may not work, however, where a large number of abnormal sperm are present.

Now IVF and similar techniques, such as GIFT, offer new hope for sub-fertile men (see page 40 for full details). Far fewer sperm are needed to achieve fertilisation *in vitro*, as the sperm do not have to make their arduous journey through the vagina, cervix, womb and tubes, with most being left behind at one stage or another. Sometimes sperm are capable of fertilising an egg but not of penetrating the cervix or surviving long in the woman's reproductive tract. By mixing sperm directly with the egg, as in IVF, these problems may be overcome. A new technique which may offer hope is intra-cytoplasmic sperm injection, ICSI, where a single sperm is injected into the egg.

Self-help

Some men can improve sperm counts with a healthier diet, stopping or reducing smoking and drinking alcohol, avoiding hot baths and not wearing tight underwear. Since the testes are very sensitive to heat, men who work in a very hot environment may experience a reduced fertility.

Sperm counts can also be lowered by illness, especially involving a fever, and may be reduced for some time afterwards since it takes three months for sperm to be produced in the body. Fortunately, this is a short-term problem that will resolve itself.

If the sperm count is consistently so low that conception is very unlikely, the main alternative with male infertility is artificial insemination by donor or donor insemination (DI). This is not a cure for infertility, but it does enable a woman with an infertile partner to conceive and bear a child. In DI, semen donated by an anonymous donor, which has been screened to ensure that it does not contain any infectious diseases, is introduced via a tube into the woman's vagina close to the cervix by a doctor or nurse. Donors are carefully screened and there is usually an attempt to match the donor's physical characteristics with that of the woman's partner. The woman goes to the clinic once a month at the most fertile time in her cycle – this is usually worked out with temperature charts. If her periods are irregular, she may be given ovulation-inducing drugs so that the doctors will be able to predict the best time for insemination. The woman is usually advised to lie on her back for about half-an-hour to enable the sperm to swim through into the womb.

Rates of conception with DI seem to be about the same as with ordinary sexual intercourse.

Going through the tests and treatments already described is in itself a remarkable testament to most couple's desire for a child they can call their own. By the time these couples come to consider the new assisted reproduction techniques, they have probably already been through months or years of tests and the more orthodox fertility treatments. At the same time, it can be difficult to call a halt. 'You feel you've already invested so many years and so much pain in all this, you just have to go on to the end,' said one woman undergoing fertility treatment.

In vitro fertilisation

Of all the new fertility treatments that have been developed, IVF has had the most impact. Since the dramatic news of the birth of baby Louise Brown on 25 July 1978, IVF has given new hope to women who previously had no hope of a baby due to blocked or scarred Fallopian tubes. At the same time, it is important to remember that IVF is demanding in time and emotional stress, is expensive, is not readily available, especially through the NHS, and the failure rate is still very high.

The success rate of IVF varies, but the most accurate figures show that just over ten per cent of all treatments actually resulted in a live baby. In specialist centres where larger numbers of IVF treatments are performed, the success rate is higher than in small centres, and the success rates also depend on the age of the women treated. If the treatment is at least a partial success – for example, the embryo may be fertilised and divide normally but fail to implant, or the woman might have an early miscarriage – most centres will probably give the woman another chance, but few recommend more than three or four attempts. The success rate of IVF also decreases with the woman's age, especially once a woman reaches the age of 39. Official figures show that live birth rates per cycle went from 16 per cent of women aged 25–34, to 11 per cent of women aged 35–39, to 5 per cent of women aged 40–44. When donated eggs were used, the figures were higher. Because older women have a lower chance of success, some IVF units will not treat women over 40.

IVF is a lengthy process. First, the woman's menstrual cycle has to be controlled with drugs such as clomiphene or HMG (Pergonal or Humagon) to ensure that she will ovulate at the right time for treatment. Drugs are usually used to stimulate her ovaries to produce more eggs or super ovulate – the woman's hormone levels have to be carefully monitored by blood tests and often by ultrasound scanning. This is done so that several eggs can be fertilised, increasing the chance of success. Also, more than one embryo may be transferred, to increase the chance of at least one implanting and developing further.

The woman then goes into hospital for an egg retrieval operation, which involves a local and sedation anaesthesia. A gas is pumped into her abdomen and an instrument called a laparoscope is introduced through a small incision in her abdomen to view the ovaries and to remove any ripe eggs from the follicles. Nowadays vaginal egg collection is sometimes done. The retrieved eggs are kept in a special culture fluid to allow them to mature. Then they are fertilised with the husband's sperm, which he is expected to produce by masturbation. Fresh semen is used if possible, as this increases the chance of success slightly, but under the stress of the procedure some men are unable to produce any. For this reason, sometimes semen is collected earlier and frozen in readiness for use at the appropriate time.

The sperm and eggs are mixed in the special culture solution to aid fertilisation. If it does take place, the embryos are allowed to develop for two to three days, to enable doctors to check that the development is normal. The embryos are then introduced into the woman's womb in a process usually referred to as embryo transfer. When the eggs are ready to be transferred, the woman will have to lie on her back with legs raised while the doctor passes a sterile catheter containing the culture fluid and embryos through the cervix (neck of the womb). This procedure is usually controlled with ultrasound. A mild sedative may be given to help the woman relax during this procedure, as passing anything through the cervix can be quite uncomfortable. Following the transfer, most women are asked to rest in bed for 10–30 minutes before leaving the clinic.

If there is a choice of good embryos available, only the best will be introduced; if not, some embryos which appear less suitable may be used, as they do sometimes develop normally and produce a healthy baby. Most abnormal embryos are lost very early; there is no evidence that babies born through IVF are any more likely to be abnormal than those conceived naturally.

Over a period of months or years, attempts to conceive with the help of IVF can take over a couple's life. For the woman, it can be very difficult to keep a job or do anything else while IVF is being attempted. The frequent disappointments can seem overwhelming. Many mothers also find that the existence of IVF makes it harder to 'let go' and accept their childlessness, or, if they already have one child, that their child will never have a brother or sister.

GIFT uses much of the same technology as IVF but is a newer and simpler procedure. In GIFT the eggs and sperm are collected in the same way as in IVF but then together are re-introduced into the Fallopian tube, via the womb, in a similar process to embryo transfer, where it is hoped that fertilisation will take place naturally. It does not require sophisticated equipment for embryo culture and the embryo is formed not in a culture medium but in the woman's own tubal fluid. This may mean that there is a greater chance of the embryo developing normally and implanting.

GIFT can only be used when the woman still has one functioning Fallopian tube, so is not an alternative to IVF. It is normally used when there is no reason found for infertility – unexplained infertility – or when there is evidence that the woman's cervix is hostile to the man's sperm, or that the sperm are failing to make it to the egg. In cases of male infertility IVF is probably preferable, and IVF is usually performed instead if there is a negative post-coital test. Success rates of 25–30 per cent have been claimed, but in reality the success rate is likely to be similar to that of IVF.

Some experts feel that GIFT is used too often in couples with unexplained infertility, who have no signs of abnormal disease and might conceive normally. One example is Jenny, who had her first son at the age of 33. Two years later they decided to try for another baby but seven months later, when nothing had happened, they went for fertility tests. Her husband Tom was told his sperm count was on the low side, but after he had given up alcohol, tried acupuncture and generally improved his level of fitness, they were told that there wasn't a problem. 'All the time there was hope; after all, we had had Peter.

'Time was getting on; Peter was four, I was nearly 38, and still no baby. We were aware that the NHS wouldn't offer treatment over the age of 40 so I felt under pressure. We tried GIFT, but this was very invasive, stressful and didn't work. My whole life was taken up with treatment and worrying about having a second baby and I felt Peter was missing out. Once I had passed 40 I decided quite simply to give up. Soon after I did so I found I was pregnant with Martin, who was born safely when I was 41. Who knows whether I might have got pregnant sooner if we hadn't been messing around with GIFT.'

Because most infertility treatments do become less successful with age, many doctors and clinics will not treat women over the age of 40. However, some doctors strongly disagree with this policy and will treat women regardless of age if they believe that the woman has a strong case and that there is no reason why she shouldn't have a baby. One of these is Professor Ian Craft, who has done pioneering work on infertility treatment but whose sometimes controversial and outspoken approach has caused him to be at odds with other members of the medical profession and with the regulatory body, the Human Fertilisation and Embryology Authority, which sets guidelines for infertility treatments and licences centres which carry out IVF and other new fertility treatments.

Professor Craft believes very strongly that older women are being discriminated against in this country by fertility specialists. One issue which he feels strongly about is the reduction of the upper limit to the number of embryos which can be transferred in IVF to three. In women over 40, whose eggs are of poorer quality – producing poorer quality embryos which are less likely to divide normally, implant, and succeed in establishing a pregnancy – transferring only three embryos considerably reduces their chances of getting pregnant, and this policy has meant their chances of getting pregnant today are less than they were in 1987. It is the fear of inducing multiple births in older women which has lead to this situation; but Craft points out that the risk of a multiple pregnancy in this age group is low; 'To my knowledge, there have never been quads in a woman over 40.'

If a woman cannot use her own eggs because the chance of pregnancy is too low, she may well succeed with donor eggs. This leads to a situation where a woman may have a child which is genetically not her own rather than one who is. When donor eggs are used, the embryos are likely to be of better quality and more likely to implant, and here the risks of a multiple pregnancy in an older age woman are very real.

The new treatment of using egg donation in women who have had premature menopause or indeed menopausal women up to the age of 50 was first used in Britain in 1986. The first mother gave birth to twins at the age of 46, the second was 43. Research has shown that provided a woman has no problems with her uterus and that it responds well to the hormone replacement therapy given, the success rate following egg donation can be high; at Professor Craft's London Gynaecology and Fertility Centre in 1993, 48 per cent of women receiving egg donation from younger women became pregnant.

The success rate when donor eggs are used seems to depend more on the age of the donor than the woman who receives the egg. In particular, miscarriage rates are the same for those of younger women rather than the higher rates usually found in older mothers.

Following the success of egg donation in helping women in their forties to conceive, other doctors – notably

Professor Severino Antinori in Rome and Dr Mark Sauer at the University of Southern California – have used the same treatment on women in their fifties with great success. In Britain, between August 1991 and November 1993, 19 women over the age of 50 had babies, either through egg donation or IVF with their own eggs; the oldest was 52. However, a survey of 61 fertility clinics to which two-thirds responded showed that three wouldn't treat women over 40, and that most refused to treat women over 45. Only four said they would treat women up to 50.

The oldest mother in Britain gave birth to twins in January 1994 at the age of 59 following treatment in Italy by Antinori. Many doctors have criticised his treatment for older women as 'irresponsible'. Professor Robert Winston, who runs the infertility clinic at the Hammersmith Hospital, told Professor Antinori in a bizarre interview on British television's *The Big Story*, 'Getting a 62-year-old woman pregnant is frankly disreputable, irresponsible. It forgets that there is a risk to the woman . . . eventually a woman will die. I think the children will also be very severely disadvantaged.' Antinori refused to take part in any kind of rational discussion.

Test tube baby pioneer Professor Robert Edwards was quoted in the *Financial Times* as saying, 'Between 50 and 60 the medical risks to mother and child are no greater than those of a younger woman, with proper care . . . Individual liberties here are being threatened. I see no reason why a woman of 60 should not have a baby. I don't know if I would go to 70 or not.'

Many criticise the treatment because it overturns the 'natural' order – although we know that it can be natural for a woman to conceive as late as 57. But how many women will want to choose such an option? The 59-year-old British woman is quoted as having delayed child bearing for career reasons. Women who have suffered infertility problems for years and given up the hope of ever having a baby may now be able to step forward and receive help. This was the case with Giuseppina Maganuco, a 54-year-old housewife from Sicily, who had spent years unsuccessfully trying to conceive and had had surgery for blocked Fallopian tubes before being told she was too old to have a baby. Antinori used donated eggs mixed with her husband's sperm to achieve the birth of baby Anna Maria in December 1991.

Lilian Cantodori, the world's oldest mother, was 61 when she gave birth to her son Andrea. She married at 40 and failed to have children, and succeeded in receiving fertility treatment after lying about her age. Finally treatment with Antinori gave her her much wanted son. Interviewed on British television, she said: 'I am proud, I am bursting with joy, I feel young again. For me a family without children is a dead family, without joy. My husband has never had a problem . . . that is why I wanted to give him this gift of love.'

Anita Blokziel was 56 when her daughter Domelda was born. She wanted another child after the terrible tragedy of her son's murder. She feels she has a lot of time and love to give her child. 'It changed my life, of course. I'm very happy . . . I have something to live for now.'

Other women seeking this treatment have remarried and want a late baby with their new partner; this is the case of 54-year-old Jane Fonda, who has announced that she wants to try for a late baby with her new husband. Singer Joni Mitchell used the technique to enable her to have a fifth child at 52, again in a second marriage.

Using donor eggs gives rise to further ethical considerations; they have been used for various infertility treatments, where the woman has no ovaries but has a healthy womb, where her eggs are unsuitable for transfer in IVF, or where she has some genetic abnormality which she does not want passed on to her children. The act of donating eggs involves the donor going through the IVF procedure except for embryo transfer; she needs to take fertility drugs to induce her to produce more than one egg for donation, and she has to undergo a minor operation – laparotomy – to collect the eggs. Because of this she must be highly motivated – some women who have experienced infertility problems themselves donate eggs, as do the sisters, friends or other relatives of the infertile woman. Some doctors are wary of using eggs from close relatives because they fear this may cause stress in the family and confusion in the child as to his or her 'real' mother; however, unknown donors are hard to find. Recent controversy has been caused by the possibility that eggs might be collected from the ovaries of aborted foetuses to make up for the shortage of donor eggs, although this might be one way around this difficulty.

Christine became an egg donor in 1991 when her friend Jane was turned down for egg donation at a private fertility clinic. 'They told her that, at 41, she was too old and that they would only give the treatment to a younger woman on whom the chances of success were higher. This was the end of a tragic saga of fertility problems and miscarriages; she had also been turned down by adoption agencies because of her age.

'I asked her if they would do an egg donation if she found a donor and offered myself. They were reluctant; we had to bully them into it. I had to have counselling to make sure I understood what I was doing and I had to sign a piece of paper waiving all my rights over the eggs.

I had an AIDS test, and I had to have a course of ten injections and use a nasal spray every four hours or so because my cycle had to be synchronised with hers so they could use some of the eggs fresh to increase her chances.

'The injections I did myself, every morning in the bum, for ten days. I had to remember to use the nasal spray which I didn't like. I had some pain in my ovaries due to the large number of eggs that were developing. Then I went in, had another large injection and a scan – I could see they had nine eggs on one side and three on the other – and a light general anaesthetic while they harvested the eggs.

'At the time I did think about it a lot. I told myself, its not a child, its just an egg, but if Jane had got pregnant on reflection I think I would have wanted to see the child and know how he or she was getting on, especially since I knew Jane. When she failed to get pregnant I was very disappointed, for her and for myself, because I had been through something quite big. She did want me to try again but I didn't want to do it; its going through too much and it isn't pleasant; I told her at the outset I'd do it once and that was all. It also stirred up a lot of emotions in the family. My mother said she was relieved not to have another grandchild out there she'd never see, and now I think to be honest I am a little relieved myself.'

Surrogate motherhood

One option for the older mother who is unable to conceive a child herself, or who perhaps has abnormalities of the womb which mean she cannot carry a child, is surrogate motherhood. Since the enormous publicity given to the first surrogate mothers, Kim Cotton in Britain and the famous 'Baby M' case in the States, where the Sterns commissioned Mary Beth Whitehead to have a baby for them and she changed her mind and took the baby back, a small number of surrogate mothers have continued to have babies for infertile women. Sometimes the surrogate mother is a friend or relative of the infertile woman, although occasionally money does change hands (though commercial surrogacy is illegal). Since the Human Fertilisation and Embryology Committee made it clear that surrogacy could be legal, some fertility specialists have used surrogate mothers, either for full surrogacy – where the infertile woman's egg is fertilised by her partner's sperm and introduced into the surrogate mother's womb – or partial surrogacy, where the surrogate mother's egg is used. Surrogacy is perhaps more common when the infertile woman is older and her chances of achieving a pregnancy in any other way are slim.

Adoption

Adoption is the main alternative path to motherhood for those who cannot have their own baby.

Older mothers, however, face very little chance of adopting a baby in this country. In 1991 fewer than 900 adoptions of babies took place soon after the birth in Britain, and most of these went to younger parents. Most adoption agencies set an upper age limit of 35 or even 30 on couples they consider to adopt a baby. The main reason given is that since the adopted child has already lost one set of parents, the chances of them losing a second set should be minimised. However, for parents in their late thirties or early forties this doesn't seem a real risk.

Recently the government published a white paper on adoption which stated that while it is 'Important that authorities and agencies should satisfy themselves that adopters have a reasonable expectation of retaining health and vigour to care for a child until he or she is grown up', there is, however, concern that some have been 'too restrictive'. It states that: 'Parents in their forties may well have much to bring to the care and upbringing of adopted children.'

Some older parents, unable to adopt in Britain, have adopted from overseas where there may be large numbers of babies and young children in orphanages, and the laws of the countries from which they adopt may be less restrictive. One such is Barbara Mostyn, who is an infertility counsellor and has been very active in STORK, the association for people who have adopted from abroad. Barbara, a single mother, adopted her son and daughter from India when she was in her mid-forties. She was also involved in researching a study of intercountry adoptions for the International Bar Association, which found that of the 210 couples involved in the study, the average age of the women was 42, with the men being several years older.

'Intercountry adoption was often a last hope for infertile couples because of the age restrictions here.' Barbara feels that because there are so many other issues involved in intercountry adoption, age is not high on the agenda. 'I had fostered a ten-year-old girl before adopting my two, and the agency had made much of my being a more mature person who knew where I was going. I'm sure they had found they'd had better luck with placing children with people in their forties. When I adopted the younger ones nobody ever mentioned my age, though this was seven years ago and things may have changed now. Personally I think there is a lot to be said for being more mature as a parent, you've got a lot of other stuff behind you and you're ready to devote yourself to the child.'

Despite the lack of babies for adoption, there are many thousands of older children in local authority care available for adoption and seeking families. While many of them show behavioural problems and have had unhappy and disrupted childhoods, many parents who do adopt them find great fulfilment in the challenge of meeting these childrens' needs and sharing in the joys and heartaches of parenthood.

3

Pregnant at last

Many women who have spent some time considering pregnancy want to make sure that they are in the best of health and have done everything possible to ensure they have a healthy child. Older women in particular may be anxious to do everything they can to offset the possible risks in being an older mother. There are some practical steps which you can take in advance to prepare yourself for the healthiest possible pregnancy.

It's important before you start trying to conceive to check that you are immune to rubella (German measles) which can cause your baby to be born blind, deaf or otherwise handicapped. If you are not immune, you can be vaccinated against rubella before you conceive. It is also a good idea to check whether you may be carrying any sexually transmitted disease. Hard to diagnose infections of pathogens such as chlamydia, gardnerella, and mycoplasma may be implicated in miscarriage and premature delivery. Blood tests for viruses such as cytomegalovirus which can cause abnormalities in the baby may also be worthwhile.

Stopping contraception

If you have been relying on an IUD, you will need to have it removed by a doctor before you conceive. As soon as an IUD is removed, you can get pregnant. If you get pregnant by chance with an IUD in place it does carry risks for mother and baby. You are more likely to have an ectopic pregnancy – a pregnancy which occurs outside the womb, usually in the Fallopian tubes – and there is a high risk of miscarriage. As many as 60 per cent of such pregnancies end before term, and the miscarriages are also more likely to occur in the second three months of pregnancy. IUDs are usually removed while you have a period, as the cervix is then slightly dilated and this aids removal.

If you have been taking the contraceptive pill, it is now advised that you stop taking it for two or three months before you wish to conceive. You can use a barrier method such as the sheath or diaphragm or natural family planning (rhythm method) during this time, although you are unlikely to use natural family planning effectively if you have not spent some time learning the technique and observing your menstrual cycle. Studies have shown that women who have taken the pill inadvertently in early pregnancy are in fact running only the very slightest extra risk of having an abnormal baby or pregnancy, and that those who conceive as soon as they stop taking the pill face no extra risk. But it is a wise precaution to make sure that your body is free of all drugs before you get pregnant. It also helps to date the pregnancy if you have had one or two normal menstrual cycles before you conceive and allows for good pregnancy care.

There is, however, some evidence that women who conceive while using spermicides, whether on their own or in combination with the diaphragm, cap or sheath, run a slightly increased risk of having a miscarriage (and, incidentally, also a greater chance of having a girl). It is obviously better to conceive when there are no traces of spermicide in the vagina. If you intend to try to conceive, it may be a good idea to ask your GP to do a cervical smear and perhaps to take a swab to check that you do not have any vaginal infection such as thrush before you get pregnant. This will usually be done at your first hospital appointment when you are pregnant, anyway, but some women prefer not to have a vaginal examination in early pregnancy, especially if they have had a miscarriage or threatened miscarriage in the past. It also makes sense to clear up any infection before rather than after a pregnancy has begun.

Avoiding drugs in pregnancy

Most women are aware that taking any drugs – including tobacco and alcohol – during pregnancy can have a harmful effect on the growing and developing baby. This is especially important in the first three months, when the baby is actually forming, as this is the time when any abnormalities would occur. Women and their partners who are planning a pregnancy, therefore, need to think about giving up smoking and cutting down drinking, ensuring that their diet contains all the elements necessary for the baby's healthy growth, and stopping any unnecessary medication. Any woman taking drugs essential for her health, for diabetes, epilepsy or high blood pressure, for example, should discuss this matter very carefully with her doctor.

Older mothers are more likely than younger ones to have

an underlying health problem, and if this is the case then you need to find out what the best options are for you before you get pregnant. Some drugs will be essential for your health, but carry a small risk of affecting the baby; this was the case with Sheila:

'I suffer from epilepsy, and I was told that it was important to continue taking my drugs, as a fit during pregnancy can be very harmful to the baby. I was told that there was a very small risk of it causing an abnormality, such as cleft palate or harelip; but in the event, Thomas was born perfect and healthy.'

There is evidence that heavy smoking or drinking on the part of the father before conception can affect the quantity and quality of his sperm, and certain drugs may also affect sperm production, so some men may need to think about this too. Sperm production takes about three months, so the father should also be thinking about changing some of his habits three or four months before you plan to get pregnant.

Alcohol

There has been a lot of controversy about the effect of taking alcohol during pregnancy, and a number of studies have been done. There is now no doubt that heavy drinking in pregnancy can have very serious effects on the baby, at its worst causing what is known as the foetal alcohol syndrome. Such babies have low birth weight, and do not catch up as do the babies of malnourished mothers or babies who have not been receiving enough nourishment in the womb. Their head circumference is smaller, and there is often mental retardation. Some have odd facial characteristics and there is a higher incidence of congenital heart disease and other abnormalities. The greater the level of alcohol drunk by the mother, the more severe the abnormalities are likely to be, and the greater the risk of the baby being miscarried or stillborn.

The situation for mothers who are moderate social drinkers is less clear, although there does appear to be evidence that women who do not drink at all in pregnancy are less likely to have miscarriages or low birth weight babies. However, the first three months appear to be the crucial time, during which the abnormalities associated with the foetal alcohol syndrome may occur. Doctors and health experts are now advising that women do not drink at all in pregnancy, and probably the best thing is to give up all alcohol when you are trying to conceive and not drink at all in the first three to four months of pregnancy, or indeed for the whole nine months. For most older women keen to have a healthy baby, this won't seem too much of a hardship.

Cigarettes

Smoking in pregnancy is very clearly linked to a higher risk of miscarriage and to low birth weight. There is some recent evidence to link congenital abnormalities with smoking, and the risk of the baby being stillborn or dying in the first few weeks of life is definitely greater. Babies are also much more likely to be born prematurely.

If you are a smoker, the best time to stop is before you get pregnant. However, giving up is not necessarily that easy. Women who smoke do so for reasons which are important to them. Some women say it helps them to relax, others that it keeps their weight down. The older you are, the more at risk you are from smoking, so its doubly important to give up. Many women find that the best way to give up smoking is to substitute something else in its place. If you smoke to relieve stress, you can try yoga for relaxation, or some other form of exercise. If your weight really is a problem, make sure that you read all the advice about the importance of diet in pregnancy. Following this should make sure you do not gain any unnecessary pounds. If your partner smokes, try to stop together – his moral support will boost your will-power and set the scene for a smoke-free household when the baby arrives. Or find a friend who also wants to stop smoking and give each other positive support.

Painkillers

Aspirin is probably the most commonly used of all drugs, and in fact its use is so common that many people do not take it seriously as a drug at all. Aspirin is known to cross the placenta into the baby's bloodstream, but its effects on the baby are not really known. Some studies, however, have shown that aspirin in large quantities may increase the risk of miscarriage in the first three months and have other harmful effects later on, so you should use aspirin sparingly in pregnancy.

Paracetamol is known to affect the liver and kidneys if taken in large quantities and could affect the developing foetus, so again should be used only sparingly in pregnancy.

Tranquillizers

There has been evidence that some tranquillizers cause an increase in birth defects, notably in cleft lip and palate. The evidence is not clear, but wherever possible tranquillizers should be avoided during pregnancy, especially in the first three months.

Antibiotics

Some antibiotics are known to be safe in pregnancy; others are definitely harmful. Penicillin is thought to be safe;

tetracycline causes yellow discolouration of the baby's teeth and may affect the growth of bones and teeth; streptomycin may be linked to deafness. You should always make sure any doctor prescribing antibiotics for you is aware that you are pregnant.

Hormonal drugs

The evidence shows that women who have taken the contraceptive pill inadvertently early in pregnancy are not at any substantial risk of affecting the baby; women who used post-coital hormonal contraception which failed also do not seem to be at risk.

Other hormonal drugs given early in pregnancy, however, do have very definite harmful effects. Hormones given in some kinds of pregnancy tests (now withdrawn from the market) caused baby girls to develop male characteristics. A drug called DES (diethylstilboestrol), given early in pregnancy to prevent miscarriage *is* now known to be linked to a rare vaginal cancer in babies born to these mothers, together with some abnormalities of the internal sex organs. Other hormones, such as progestogens, given in pregnancy to prevent miscarriage or for other problems, may have harmful effects and are best avoided, although there is no conclusive evidence to prove this. In some cases where a woman has miscarried because of low hormone levels, this treatment may be justified.

Anti-nausea drugs

The use of anti-nausea drugs in pregnancy is very controversial. Thalidomide was given to women to prevent sickness in early pregnancy and shocked the world by the horrific abnormalities it caused. Other drugs have been used to prevent nausea and vomiting in the first three months of pregnancy, but most of these have also been eventually withdrawn because of a possible link with birth defects (Debendox is one).

Because the baby is so very vulnerable to drugs in the first three months of pregnancy when nausea occurs, taking any kind of drug must be viewed as a last resort, and anyone who can possibly manage without drugs would be well advised to. However, getting the support to do so may not be easy.

'I had terrible nausea and vomiting in both my pregnancies. In the second pregnancy it was worse, and lasted from five weeks (that was how I knew I was pregnant) to 16. I felt sick every minute of the day, and I was sick frequently – two or three times some days, only once on others. It wasn't just in the morning, it was all the time and was worse when I didn't eat regular, small snacks and meals. At around seven or eight weeks I had 48 hours when I couldn't keep anything down, and because I had an active toddler to look after, I was getting desperate. I rang the doctor who suggested an anti-nausea drug. I was tempted, but in the end I said "no". In fact, the vomiting did get better after that acute phase and I did manage to eat, though I lost weight over the first three months. After 16 weeks it got dramatically better and I was so pleased that I got through without drugs. I know I would have been worried for the rest of the pregnancy that there would be something wrong with the baby if I'd taken anything. I wish doctors would help give you confidence to go without drugs unless you really can't keep anything down at all.'

Some women do experience such severe nausea that they are only able to get through this phase with the help of medication. Ranu was shocked to discover she was pregnant with twins at the age of 39 (older mothers have a greater chance of twin pregnancies; see page 77). 'I was expecting twin boys and I was so sick in the first two months I couldn't even keep down a glass of water, so in the end I took Debendox (this was before it was withdrawn). There was nothing wrong with the twins at all, they are fantastic, perfect. I just couldn't have carried on without it.'

There are, however, alternatives to drugs, including herbal drinks or homoeopathic remedies which some women find help with nausea and vomiting. But the best way to cope with nausea and vomiting seems to be careful attention to diet, which should consist of nutritious foods such as wholemeal bread, fresh fruit, nuts, raisins and dried fruit, raw vegetables, cereals; wholemeal biscuits and muesli bars can be good if you want something sweet. Eating small, frequent amounts helps. Fatty or very sweet foods are likely to make you feel worse rather than better, and you should avoid spicy food, alcohol, or cigarette smoke. If preparing food makes you feel ill, get someone else to do it for you if at all possible, or have meals that need the minimum preparation. Drink plenty of (mainly fresh) fruit juices, herbal teas and water; avoid tea and coffee – and many people find milky drinks make sickness worse, too. Remember to keep on eating regardless. It is much more unpleasant being sick on an empty stomach than a full one, and starving yourself is likely to make the nausea much worse. Even if food stays in the stomach only a short time, some goodness will have been absorbed.

Alternative medicine such as homeopathy or acupuncture may be able to help. You may also try some specially designed elastic bands covered with soft material which are worn around the wrists to put pressure on certain points; these are supposed to help relieve travel or morning sickness.

Diet during pregnancy

Maintaining a healthy diet during pregnancy is the best thing you can do for yourself and for your baby. Junk food can be harmful in pregnancy because it does not provide enough of the vitamins and nutrients needed by the growing baby; it is also high in salt and other additives which increase stress on the liver and kidneys, which, in turn, have to eliminate the salt from the body. If you eat the right foods, you won't need to worry about taking vitamin supplements; you should be careful of taking large quantities of vitamin supplements as some vitamins, notably vitamin A, can be harmful if taken in excess. Also, if you eat healthily you won't need to worry about whether you're putting on the right amount of weight or not; your body will do that automatically.

Weight gain

It is normal to gain weight in pregnancy and most of this appears during the second three months. The increased weight will be the weight of the baby, the placenta, the waters surrounding the baby, increased fluid and tissue in the breasts as they prepare to produce milk, and a greater quantity of blood circulating in the body. Some women also experience fluid retention which will adjust after the baby is born.

A normal weight gain during pregnancy is 20–30 lb (9–13.5 kg). Some women gain less, others more, without there being any need for alarm. If you are planning to breast feed your baby, you should also remember that you will be laying down some stores of fat to feed your new baby and that the pounds will roll off as you produce your milk. Doctors used to worry a lot about 'excessive' weight gain in pregnancy as this can put an extra strain on the body, making high blood pressure and cardiovascular problems more likely. However, this in itself was a reaction to the exhortations previously made to women to 'eat for two'. But aiming for the other extreme and trying to stay slim in pregnancy is equally harmful.

It is particularly damaging to try to diet and lose weight in pregnancy unless your are overweight and under medical supervision, as you may be denying the baby vital nourishment. Again, eating the right food is the key. If you eat well you will feel well, be less inclined to want to 'fill up' on sweet things, and your body will gain and shed weight naturally during and after the pregnancy.

A healthy diet

A healthy diet means eating a balanced combination of proteins, carbohydrates, fats and vitamins. This can be achieved by eating reasonable quantities of fresh meat and fish, eggs, pasteurised cheese and milk, fresh fruits and vegetables, wholemeal bread and cereals. Fresh green vegetables in particular are full of the minerals and vitamins needed by your body and that of the growing foetus. Avoid foods which have 'empty' calories, such as highly refined sugary cakes and sweet fizzy drinks, biscuits, salty foods which will encourage fluid retention, and drinks such as coffee, tea and cocoa, as well as wine, spirits and beer.

What you need and why

Protein
Proteins contain the basic building blocks that make up your body and are absolutely vital in pregnancy for the

baby to grow and develop. Your protein requirements increase by about 50 per cent during pregnancy. The best sources of protein are meat and fish, dairy products, eggs, and in pulses and some green vegetables – lentils, peas, beans, seeds, nuts and yeast are all very rich in protein. If you are a vegetarian you can still get enough protein from the latter, but some vegetarian women choose to eat a little fish and chicken in pregnancy to boost their protein intake. Fish is particularly valuable, as it contains a lot of minerals and vitamins and is also low in fat.

Carbohydrates

Carbohydrates are vital in meeting your energy needs in pregnancy. They do not have to be fattening: potatoes, especially if baked in their jackets, are not fattening and also contain a lot of vitamin C. Bread, flour, cereals and root vegetables are all good sources of carbohydrate, and it's best not to skip these; you may then feel hungry again and fill up on sweet things instead.

Fat

You do not need extra fat in pregnancy, and if you are gaining excessive weight you can cut down on butter, oils and sauces and have low-fat yoghurts and curd cheese. However, you will need to make sure you are not missing out on the fat-soluble vitamins.

Minerals

A number of minerals are known to be essential for health, especially during pregnancy. Because the body's blood volume increases so much, there is an extra demand for iron in pregnancy, and this is especially true in second and subsequent pregnancies, particularly if there has not been a long gap since the last baby was born. You can increase iron in the blood by eating iron-rich foods, notably dark green vegetables such as spinach and watercress, offal such as liver (some mothers may be advised to avoid liver altogether) and kidneys, egg yolks, whole grains, pulses and nuts, and nut spreads such as peanut butter. Your haemoglobin levels will be checked in pregnancy to make sure that you are not getting anaemic; if you are, iron pills can be prescribed. Calcium is important in pregnancy for the formation of bones and teeth and to ensure blood clotting. Milk and dairy foods are a good source, but so are vegetables, whole grains, pulses and nuts. Spinach, rhubarb and cocoa help prevent the absorption of calcium, so do not have too much of these foods. Potassium, zinc and other trace elements are also important. Seafood is a good source of many minerals and oysters are particularly rich in zinc.

Fibre
Many women find that they tend to become constipated in pregnancy, as the pregnancy hormones slow down the movement of the muscles of the bowel. Constipation can make mothers feel unwell, as well as leading to piles (haemorrhoids) if you are constantly straining to pass motions. It is important to eat foods which have plenty of fibre, such as wholemeal bread, unrefined cereals like muesli or those which are rich in bran, and raw fruit and vegetables, and to drink a lot of fluids.

Vitamins
Vitamins are essential in pregnancy, both to keep you healthy and for the development of your baby. Research has shown that mothers who are short of certain vitamins are at a greater risk of having a handicapped baby or a

Nutrient	Rich sources	Good sources	What it does
Vitamin A	Egg yolk, oily fish, whole milk, butter, carrots	Liver, kidney, green and yellow vegetables	Helps resist infection, essential for vision, keeps hair etc. in good condition.
Vitamin B1 Thiamine	Wheatgerm, nuts, pork	Oatmeal, liver, kidney, peas, wholemeal bread	Aids digestion, necessary for growth.
Vitamin B2 Riboflavin	Brewer's yeast, wheatgerm	Green vegetables, milk, eggs, liver	Builds brain cells, prevents infections and bleeding gums.
Niacin	Beef extract, liver, peanuts, salmon, sardines	Kidney, cooked meats, mackerel, other fish	Prevents eye and skin problems, essential for normal growth and development.
Vitamin B6 Pyridoxine	Yeast, liver, kidney, mackerel	Meat, fish, eggs, banana, pineapple, wholemeal bread	Deficiency causes disease of the nerves and anaemia.
Vitamin B12	Liver, pilchards, sardines, herring	Tongue, turkey, tuna, salmon, beef, lamb, egg	Necessary to form red blood cells and nervous system.
Folic acid	Liver, dark green vegetables	Kidney, peanuts, walnuts, wheatgerm, eggs, lettuce, mushroom, tomatoes, oranges	As vitamin B12. Deficiency linked to spina bifida.

Nutrient	Rich sources	Good sources	What it does
Vitamin C Ascorbic Acid	Blackcurrants, strawberries, broccoli, sprouts, cabbage	Oranges, lemons, broad beans, asparagus	Helps iron absorption, important for healing.
Calcium	Milk, hard cheese	Small whole fish, especially shellfish, soya flour, figs, peanuts, walnuts	Essential for healthy bones and teeth.
Iron	Liver, black sausage, kidney, beef, soya, oysters	Lamb, chicken, turkey, ham	Essential for formation of red blood cells.
Zinc	Oysters, wheatgerm, wheat bran	Beef, lamb, liver, cheese, milk, oatmeal, wholegrain cereals	Helps form many enzymes and proteins.

Table 3.1

baby who is born with low birth weight. Table 3.1 shows which vitamins you need and what they do. Remember that taking too much of certain vitamins can be harmful too, so check with your doctor.

Folic acid – a B group vitamin – has been found to help prevent spina bifida and other neural tube defects, so it can be a good idea to supplement your diet with this if you are likely to be short of this vitamin.

Foods to avoid

Recently publicity has been given to a number of foods which may contain micro-organisms that can cause harmful disease in pregnancy. Listeriosis is an illness caused by a bacteria, listeria monocytogenes. Listeriosis is a mild, flu-like disease in adults, but in a pregnant woman it can cause miscarriage, stillbirth, or severe illness in the newborn baby. Listeria can be found in soft cheeses such as Brie, Camembert and blue-veined cheeses, and can also be found in patés. Ready-cooked meals can also contain low quantities of listeria and must therefore be very thoroughly heated. Salmonella, which can cause acute food poisoning, may be found in undercooked chicken and in raw or soft-boiled eggs, so some women prefer to avoid these. Recent research has shown high levels of vitamin A are concentrated in liver, and this can be harmful, so don't overdo the eating of liver as an iron source.

Toxoplasmosis is another organism which causes only mild symptoms in an adult but which can injure the foetus, causing blindness or hydrocephalus which can cause brain damage. Toxoplasmosis is found in some raw meat, unpasteurised goat's milk or cheese, unwashed raw fruit and vegetables, and in anything contaminated by cat faeces.

Since a pregnancy is not usually confirmed till six or eight weeks, and it may take a little time for the body to build up depleted stores of vitamins and essential minerals, it is very important to adjust your diet before you become pregnant if at all possible. A good diet will also make you feel stronger and healthier and help you through the demanding months of pregnancy, through the birth itself, and through the post-natal period. It will help you to enjoy your baby, too.

Preconceptual care

As more is known about how diet, drugs and other substances in the environment might affect the unborn baby more and more mothers are trying to prepare well in advance for the birth of their baby. Genetic counsellors are available through the NHS if there is any genetic disorder in the family or if you are at greater risk of having a handicapped baby. Advice on diet and general health care in pregnancy may be given at your antenatal clinic.

It is worth having your health checked before you conceive. You might like to have a smear test carried out. You can also have a swab done to check that there are no harmful micro-organisms in the vagina; recent research has shown that thrush and gardnerella, a bacteria which causes bacterial vaginosis, may be linked to a difficulty to conceive, that an organism called mycoplasma may be linked to miscarriage and gardnerella to premature deliveries. Not all such infections cause symptoms, but may flare up or cause problems in pregnancy. So checking before you're pregnant may be wise.

There is an organisation, Foresight, which gives information and advice to women who are planning a pregnancy. Foresight will also do tests on samples of your hair and blood to check that you are well nourished and not short of any essential vitamins or minerals. However, not all the medical information they give out is correct, and many doctors believe that the tests they do are unrealistic, and that in most cases the shortage of vitamins and minerals would not be enough to place the mother at higher risk of having an abnormal baby. It is also true that the majority of women do not want to wait months to conceive, and many conceive by accident, or experience problems in conceiving, and these mothers may feel guilty that they are not doing the right thing: 'We started out with all the best intentions, stopping smoking and drinking, taking vitamin pills and potions and eating only health-foody things without any additives. But it took me nearly two years to get pregnant. By the end I was fed up with the whole thing – we never enjoyed ourselves any more, we felt guilty about everything we ate or didn't eat. In the end I just ate what I felt like and got on with it.'

Genetic counselling is available at many hospitals for those who are worried that they may be at extra risk of having a handicapped baby – this includes older mothers and those who have some hereditary illness or defect in their family.

'We had genetic counselling at the hospital because I was 40, my husband was in his forties too, and his child by his previous marriage had had problems – her gullet and windpipe were joined and there was a blockage to the entrance to her stomach. She had to be operated on at birth, although she's fine now. We were told that this could be picked up on the ultrasound scan, as the baby would not be able to swallow the amniotic fluid which would otherwise show up in the stomach – this was very reassuring as we would want to know in advance so the baby could be born where they would be geared up to do immediate surgery. I was also concerned about the extra risk of having a Down's syndrome baby – I was surprised at how greatly the risk went up between the ages of 40 and 41. We decided to have the amniocentesis and other tests done because we felt we couldn't have coped with a severely handicapped baby. I found the counselling very helpful and reassuring.'

Genetic counselling can be very helpful in enabling the couple to talk through any worries they have and to put the risks they are facing into proportion, and this is especially true for older mothers who may feel this pregnancy is the only chance they've got. It can also be very helpful in establishing the reasons for any previous babies born with handicaps in the family, or for several miscarriages, and point towards ways of overcoming them. For example, it has been shown that mothers of babies with spina bifida had far fewer affected babies in subsequent pregnancies if they took supplements of vitamin B and folic acid. Some couples who have had several miscarriages have been told that this is linked to a genetic problem but that if they persist there is a chance they will have a normal baby, and this has encouraged them to carry on.

Keeping fit in pregnancy

Exercise and general physical fitness are very important in pregnancy. Your body changes shape and new stresses and strains are put on it, culminating in the physical stress of the birth itself. By making sure your body is strong and fit you will be helping yourself in pregnancy and working towards an active and safe birth, as well as giving yourself energy and resilience for the demanding time ahead.

During pregnancy your joints tend to loosen slightly; this enables the pelvis to stretch during birth to let the baby through, but also means that you are more likely to strain your ligaments and joints and, especially, your back. You should be careful of putting strain on your back by picking things up awkwardly or carrying loads which are too heavy. The weight of your baby in front will make even simple movements like getting out of a chair or a bed potentially damaging for your back, so take care to move in such a way as not to put undue strain on it. Roll onto your side and sit up from there to get out of bed and use your legs, not your back, to lever yourself out of a chair. When picking up a toddler or a bag of shopping, squat down and then push up with your thighs rather than bending your back right over.

There are a number of exercises you can do in pregnancy to keep yourself supple and to strengthen muscles that you will use in the birth itself. However, not everyone is very good at doing a programme of exercises and if you are working or you have other children, it may be hard to fit them in. Gentle walking and, especially, swimming are good exercises in pregnancy if you enjoy them. You can carry on with your usual sports, but gently; remember that if you get out of breath you are depriving your baby of oxygen too. Exercise in pregnancy should be gentle rather than rushed.

Women who want an active labour should practise holding positions such as squatting, standing on all fours or sitting semi-upright to see what position they find most comfortable and to strengthen the muscles they will use.

All women, however, will benefit from locating and exercising the pelvic floor muscles which are so important in pregnancy and childbirth. These muscles support the uterus, bowel and bladder and about half of all women who have had children suffer from some weakness in these muscles, with such symptoms as discomfort in the pelvic area or leaking a little urine when they sneeze, cough or lift heavy objects. If these muscles become too weak it can lead to prolapse of the womb. You can feel what it is like to use the pelvic floor muscles by tightening your buttocks and pulling upwards as if you want to empty your bladder but must hold on. The same muscle tightens the vagina and can cause pleasant sensations when you are making love. If you cannot feel the muscles tighten, then try interrupting the flow of urine when you are emptying your bladder; you will soon be able to recognise the sensation. You can exercise these muscles unseen every day when you are lying down, standing or sitting. Simply do four to six contractions of about five seconds each at various intervals during the day. You can try to do them at the same times each day – when you're cleaning your teeth or taking a bath, washing up, and so on – to help you incorporate them in your daily routine. It is important to carry on with these exercises after the baby is born, to strengthen them after the inevitable stretching they will have received during the birth.

Antenatal care

Good antenatal care, as well as taking care of your health and looking after yourself, is the key to a healthy pregnancy. Doctors and other health professionals are aware that it is mainly through improving antenatal care that they can better the health of mothers and babies and reduce the small number of babies who are born with difficulties and who die. Much of the antenatal care you will receive is routine, but it is there to pick up any problems and take action to prevent them from getting worse. Skipping on appointments or failing to make use of the services available is putting yourself and your baby at risk, and this may be particularly so for the older mother. One study carried out by the World Health Organisation showed that older mothers (over 35) in countries where they received good antenatal care were at no greater risk during pregnancy and labour than younger women; this was not true in countries with poor health care during pregnancy.

Finding out you are pregnant

Most women will want to know that they are pregnant as soon as possible, especially if they have had problems conceiving. There are now modern pregnancy tests available which can tell you accurately whether you are pregnant or not as soon as, or even before, your period is due. These tests are available from chemists at a modest price – each packet usually contains two tests, so that if the first isn't positive, you can repeat it a few days later to make sure. Because these tests are rather more expensive than the standard test carried out by your doctor two weeks after your first missed period, they are not usually available on the NHS. You will find that if you get a pregnancy test done free through your GP, hospital or family-planning clinic, it will not normally be done until two weeks after your period is due and you will not usually have to wait for the result.

'It was silly because when my period was overdue I did a

home test and it was positive. Then they did one at Bart's (St Bartholomew's Hospital, London) and it was negative. We were both very disappointed. But my period didn't start, and I felt pregnant. So I did another home test which was positive. I rang my husband and asked him to pop home from work and check I wasn't imagining it, and he agreed it was positive. But the next test from the hospital was negative too – until the GP rang and said they had made an error. It seemed so silly that a home test was so much better than the hospital one!'

Having your pregnancy confirmed early enables you to stop drinking and take care of your diet, if you haven't already done so, and book early for your antenatal appointments. Once you know you are pregnant you should talk things over with your GP and explain any preferences you have for the kind of birth you would like, which hospitals you prefer, whether you would like a GP delivery if possible and whether you would like a home birth if that can be arranged. Your GP will know the options in the area and will be able to discuss with you what is best, and then may refer you to the system of your choice. In practice this is not always the case, and older mothers in particular may find they are only offered a hospital birth or are under strong pressure to have the baby in hospital. In some areas, too, the choice of hospital is limited. Many GPs do not do deliveries at all.

The vast majority of births now take place in hospitals and most people also have their antenatal care under the hospital. Even if you are having a hospital birth, however, you can arrange to have shared care with your GP, if he or she does obstetric care, which may mean shorter waits for appointments as well as the comfort of a familiar face. You may also be seen by a midwife at your doctor's surgery, especially if it is part of a larger health clinic. Although things seem to have improved in antenatal care, the majority of women find waiting at the hospital clinics is still a problem. There are usually no facilities for older children and toddlers. Women complain that they are seen by someone different each time and never even see the consultant they are booked under, and many women find the care impersonal and offhand. If you have any special problems, you are more likely to see the consultant, so if you just see the midwife at every visit you can console yourself with the fact that your pregnancy is progressing normally. On the whole, older mothers do not find themselves too much of an oddity at antenatal clinics.

'I realised that I could be the mother of the woman sitting next to me, but it didn't really seem to matter. We were both going through the same thing. I was never once made to feel that I was old or doing anything out the ordinary by the other women or by the hospital staff. I should think the average age of mothers at the hospital was 30–35, though this hospital does specialise in women with potential difficulties and older mothers and it is in London, which I think makes a difference. I was astounded at the number of older women – it seems that women have their careers first and then their families.'

Routine antenatal tests

You are usually booked for your first appointment at around the twelfth week of pregnancy, when your medical history will be taken, together with any details of previous pregnancies. Your height and shoe size are measured, as this gives some indication of the size of your pelvis, though women usually have babies in proportion to their own size. You are also likely to be given an internal examination to confirm the pregnancy and check the womb is the size it should be for your dates, check for any abnormalities of the pelvis and check that the cervix (neck of the womb) is tightly closed. A cervical smear is also usually taken.

If you have had a history of miscarriage it is likely that the doctor will agree not to examine you internally at this stage if you wish, though there is no particular evidence to suggest that this might provoke a miscarriage.

A blood test is also taken to find your major blood group, particularly whether you are rhesus positive or negative. About 80 per cent of the population are rhesus positive. If you are rhesus negative and your baby is rhesus positive, and it is a second or subsequent pregnancy, there is small chance that you may make sufficient antibodies to rhesus positive blood to damage your baby's blood cells. Because of this, if you are rhesus negative, blood samples will be taken at various points during your pregnancy to check on antibody levels, which only rarely become too high. Very occasionally a baby suffering from rhesus incompatibility may have to be delivered early by Caesarean section and receive an exchange transfusion.

Rhesus incompatibility is becoming rarer because most rhesus negative mothers now have an injection of anti-rhesus globulin which prevents them producing antibodies. If this is done after every delivery or abortion, future babies are safe from rhesus incompatibility.

Your haemoglobin level is checked to make sure you are not anaemic (this test will be repeated later in the pregnancy). You are also screened for German measles antibodies to check that you are immune, and for any sexually transmitted diseases.

Your breasts are usually examined at the first visit to check for any lumps. They are not being checked to see whether you can breast feed or not – whatever size or shape your breasts or nipples are, you should be able to breast feed successfully. If your nipples are inverted, there is no treatment which has been found to help antenatally, and you will still be able to breast feed; you may just need a little extra help in getting the baby to latch on properly (see page 168).

At every visit you will be weighed to check the growth of the baby and that your weight gain is satisfactory. Your urine is tested at every visit – the first time it will be screened for any infection, every other visit it will be tested for the presence of protein in the urine which could indicate you have pre-eclampsia (see below) and to check that you are not developing diabetes.

The abdomen is measured at every visit to check that the womb is growing in size according to your dates and after 20–24 weeks your baby's heartbeat can be monitored with a stethoscope or sometimes a device called a sonic aid. Your blood pressure is also measured at every visit, as high blood pressure can indicate a number of problems including pre-eclampsia, and your ankles and fingers are checked for water retention.

Pre-eclampsia or toxaemia is one condition that doctors are on the alert for in pregnancy, as it can be prevented if caught early and the risk to the unborn baby be reduced. Older mothers are at a greater risk of this condition, so it's important to keep up regular visits. The cause is unknown, although in some cases it has been linked to poor nutrition. The symptoms are water retention, causing puffiness of ankles, legs and wrists, high blood pressure, and if the condition is allowed to progress unchecked, the blood pressure rises further and the mother suffers headaches and even fits. The baby is at risk and may not be getting enough nourishment, and there is an increased risk of premature labour.

Pre-eclampsia can usually be treated by bed rest, and women suffering this condition are often admitted to hospital so that they and the baby can be monitored. Usually complete rest solves the problem, but if it does get worse, the baby may have to be born early by Caesarean section to ensure that it survives.

Twin pregnancies

It may come as a surprise to learn that older mothers are more likely to have twins than their younger counterparts. Identical twins are the result of the fertilised egg splitting in two and developing in exactly the same way, since they contain exactly the same genetic material. This occurs at random and does not seem to be influenced by heredity or age. Non-identical twins occur when two eggs are released in a cycle by the ovary, and are both fertilised. Non-identical twins are no more alike than other brothers and sisters, and the chance of having them increases with age, especially if there are other non-identical twins in the family or if a woman has been taking certain fertility drugs before conceiving.

A twin pregnancy needs special care and monitoring as it puts an extra strain on your body, and this is particularly true of older mothers. You will need to watch for high blood pressure and anaemia and will need extra rest. Twin babies are more likely to be born prematurely and sometimes one baby grows larger than the other, which may be of low birth weight – or both babies may be underweight. The birth will need to take place in hospital as there is an increased risk to the second baby if it is not born soon after the first, especially if it is not in the usual head-down position, and antenatal care will need to be particularly vigilant, since problems such as high blood pressure are more likely to occur in a twin pregnancy, especially when the mother is older.

Emotional changes in pregnancy

It is as important to take care of yourself emotionally in pregnancy as it is to take care of your physical well-being, although this is much more difficult. Many women find that they change a lot in pregnancy, that they feel more vulnerable and easily upset, or that they become preoccupied with the new life inside them and find it more difficult to keep up at work, to visit friends or to put energy into making their relationship with their partner run smoothly. Pregnancy can thus be a very testing time for many couples, though potentially a very rewarding one, too.

For older women, pregnancy and its loss of physical independence may come as something of a shock. 'I was used to being able to control everything,' says Sheila, 41, 'and then suddenly I couldn't. I thought I could carry on just the same but my body told me differently. At the beginning it was the tiredness and the nausea. At the end it was that I was just so big, and I found I just couldn't concentrate. And if anything at work went wrong, I just felt like bursting into tears. I felt so vulnerable.'

Denise became pregnant at the age of 41 after trying for two years. 'It never occurred to me that I wouldn't conceive. I assumed if I wanted a baby I could have it like everything else.' The pregnancy came at a good time, when Denise had some time off work, which helped her get through the morning sickness and tiredness. 'I think my age did make me more tired. I was working hard and trying to prove it didn't make any difference.'

A woman's feelings may depend on how well she feels in pregnancy as well as on the closeness of her relationships with her partner, family and friends and, perhaps most important of all, how much the pregnancy was planned and hoped for:

'I got pregnant by accident – I wasn't too pleased when I got the news! I had a teenage daughter by my first marriage and none in my second, but we'd agreed not to have any. My initial reaction was resentment and the doctor offered a termination – I woke up and cried every morning to think that I was pregnant. But my husband had no children in his first marriage and when I sat and thought about an abortion, I couldn't have done it because of him.'

'After infertility tests and a miscarriage I was so thrilled to be pregnant that I went around in a haze for the whole pregnancy, despite morning sickness and other discomforts. I couldn't contain myself, it was so exciting.'

Some women find work becomes a strain: 'I thought pregnancy wouldn't change me. What a hope! For the first three months I was terribly, bone-achingly tired. I couldn't concentrate on work. I hate to admit this, but it was true.'

Madeleine had the same experience. 'It was difficult staggering into work in the early months with bad morning sickness. I used to throw up regularly in the office loo as soon as I got in – the miracle was I was never sick on the bus! Then, later, I used to sit at meetings and be unable to concentrate properly because the baby was kicking so much – it seemed so odd to be there talking about work plans and schedules while this tremendous thing was going on inside me. I also became very cow-like and contented – I couldn't rush for deadlines any more, they seemed so unimportant.'

Others, perhaps those with less pressure on them, find that they can really relax and enjoy the pregnancy and live it to the full. 'I felt great when pregnant. I felt fit and healthy and relaxed and let myself be taken care of.'

Antenatal depression

A great deal has been written about postnatal depression, but very little about antenatal depression, although it is quite common for women to be depressed in some stages of pregnancy. Many women feel overwhelmingly tired and this means that social engagements, work, house-work and relationships all suffer if other people do not understand:

'I used to go to bed whenever I could, so the house got in a terrible mess because I couldn't face cleaning it. I couldn't be bothered to cook nice meals and I didn't have the energy to go out to parties or the cinema with friends. My husband used to groan because every evening about nine o'clock I'd just say, "I'm exhausted, I'm going to bed now". A lot of the time I was too tired for sex as well.'

Depression is perhaps particularly common in a second pregnancy, especially when the woman has a toddler or young child to care for, and/or is working. No one makes quite the same fuss of you after the first pregnancy and it is harder to get the extra rest you need. Again, working women may find pregnancy particularly tiring and feel that they are not being so efficient in their jobs, which again can cause feelings of depression.

Older women in pregnancy, particularly, may worry about the health of their baby and about the birth itself – whether they will have complications and whether there will be anything wrong with the baby. This may also depend on the attitude of the doctors and midwives caring for the woman in pregnancy:

'I found out I was pregnant by accident in my early-forties, too late to have an abortion or even the tests [tests dealt with in Chapter Four] – my GP was very nervous about it all and my husband worried and thought something would be wrong. The scans gave a different date to my GP and showed the baby was small – it was all a worry.

'I worried about the birth because of my age, but the consultant was fantastic. He said, "You're a healthy woman – you should have a super-easy birth" – he was very reassuring.'

Sex in pregnancy

Many couples continue with a happy and fulfilling sex life right through the pregnancy, and doctors today reassure women that sex in pregnancy is perfectly safe and will not harm the baby. There are a few circumstances in which this is not so: women who have had a history of miscarriage or threatened miscarriage may be advised to avoid sexual intercourse until after the time when the miscarriage or threat occurred, or till after the first 12–16 weeks of pregnancy. Women who have had a premature labour may also be advised to avoid intercourse in the last months, for fear of precipitating labour. Research has shown that substances called prostaglandins found in sperm can help soften the cervix and induce labour, so if your baby goes overdue sexual intercourse can be a good way of getting labour started. In a normal pregnancy, however, there is no evidence that having sexual intercourse or experiencing an orgasm will upset the pregnancy.

Many women find that they get increased pleasure from sex in pregnancy; the increased blood supply to the genital area and the strong contractions of the womb during orgasm can all heighten sensation. Some women feel a particular closeness to their partners during pregnancy which they need to express sexually and others seek reassurance that they are still desirable.

Not all women feel this, however, and some feel that they need to retreat somewhat into their bodies and concentrate on the baby, and that sex is an intrusion into this. Tiredness and other discomforts at the end of pregnancy may also make some women feel less like sex, while others may feel that different ways of expressing love and affection are more appropriate. One small study into women's feelings about sex before and after the birth showed that only half the women in the sample were still having sexual intercourse 12 weeks before the birth, so these feelings are very normal. Towards the end of pregnancy, sex in the usual positions may become very uncomfortable so it is a good idea to experiment with other positions – something which many couples find adds spice to their sex life. A lot of women find full penetration very uncomfortable at the end of pregnancy, especially when the baby's head has 'engaged' and dropped right down into the pelvis, so positions which avoid too deep penetration are preferable. It is important for women to talk openly to their partners about their wishes and feelings in pregnancy, otherwise sex can become a focus for dissatisfaction and resentment.

Problems in pregnancy

Anaemia

Women are always prone to a deficiency of iron because of the repeated blood loss of menstruation. If a woman does not have sufficient reserves before pregnancy, anaemia may result because of the increase in the volume of blood circulating through the body.

The symptoms of anaemia are tiredness, lethargy, irritability and paleness of the skin. Anaemia can easily be treated with iron supplements.

Diabetes

Diabetic women run special risks in pregnancy and will usually be kept under careful medical supervision. However, nowadays it is perfectly possible for the diabetic woman to have a normal pregnancy and labour.

Diabetes can be unmasked by pregnancy because of the extra strains put on the body, and this is more likely with an older mother. If diabetes is detected with a urine test, the mother's blood sugar levels will be monitored. Diabetes may be controlled by diet alone, or with insulin injections, the dosage of which may need to be altered as the pregnancy progresses. Because the diabetic woman has a risk of having an unusually large baby, birth is sometimes induced early or the mother may be recommended to have a Caesarean section.

Jenny is a diabetic who had two children in her thirties.

'I knew from the beginning of my first pregnancy that I was going to have a Caesarean. When my first child was born almost all diabetic women ended up with a Caesarean. It was done with an epidural so that I would be awake to see the baby, but the epidural went wrong, I had a headache and had to lie flat on my back for 48 hours after the birth and I had pains in the legs for about ten days afterwards.

'I waited five years to get pregnant again. I had myself referred to Professor Beard at St Mary's who I knew had pioneered natural childbirth for diabetics. I wanted to have a normal birth for a healthy person, as that is what I consider myself to be. There was a slight worry as the baby went overdue, but at one week late I went in and was induced and had a normal, easy birth.'

Pre-eclampsia

This is a metabolic disturbance in pregnancy with symptoms of high blood pressure, swelling of the feet, hands and ankles and protein in the urine. It occurs more frequently in older women, but is also linked to obesity and poor nutrition. If untreated, the woman will get headaches, blurred vision and may go on to develop eclampsia, in which she suffers from fits. The main risk is not to the mother but to the baby, as there is a high risk of premature labour.

Pre-eclampsia is normally treated with bed rest and sedation and a careful check is kept on the mother's blood pressure. If it is late in the pregnancy and the blood pressure rises too high, the baby will normally be delivered early by Caesarean section.

Antepartum haemorrhage

Bleeding before 28 weeks in pregnancy usually results in a miscarriage. After 28 weeks any bleeding is known as antepartum haemorrhage and has two main causes: abruptio placentae, a rare condition in which the placenta separates from the wall of the uterus, and placenta praevia. Both these conditions are slightly more common in older mothers.

Placenta praevia is a condition where the placenta is attached to the lower part of the womb, near or even over the cervix. This results in bleeding during pregnancy and more bleeding as soon as labour starts. Usually it can be picked up by an ultrasound scan. Most mothers with this condition have to rest in hospital until the baby is due, to prevent bleeding and so that the baby can be delivered by Caesarean section.

Miscarriage

One problem which is of great concern to older mothers is the risk of miscarriage. This risk is particularly worrying for mothers who have had problems in conceiving.

The risk of miscarriage for older mothers is much greater than for younger mothers. It is not commonly known that as many as one in six recognised pregnancies end in miscarriage; the numbers would be still higher if all pregnancies were counted, including those which end so soon that a period is only slightly delayed or not delayed at all. There seems to be a slightly higher risk of miscarriage in a first pregnancy.

For older mothers, though, miscarriages are even more common. One study of women who conceived through artificial insemination by donor showed that by the age of 40 a mother had a 50 per cent chance of having a miscarriage. Studies have shown that about 50 per cent of miscarried foetuses are genetically abnormal – this is why many people try to comfort the woman who has lost her baby with the fact that 'its nature's way of getting rid of abnormal babies'. In older mothers the proportion of abnormal foetuses may be higher. New research on helping older women conceive using hormone replacement and donated eggs has shown that it is more likely to be the quality of the embryo than deficiencies in the mother's womb that cause failure of pregnancy.

Having one miscarriage does not mean that there is any greater chance of having a second one. After two miscarriages, the chance does go up from about one in five to one in three; after three subsequent miscarriages the chances are about 50–50 that the pregnancy will go to term. But the great majority of women who have miscarriages will go on to have a healthy baby in the end.

Medically, a distinction is made between miscarriages which occur up to about 12 or 13 weeks, and those which occur after this time, as they usually have different causes. The great majority of miscarriages – about 85 per cent – occur before the end of the twelfth week of pregnancy.

What happens when you have a miscarriage?

The first sign of a miscarriage during the first three months of pregnancy is a small amount of bleeding, like the start of a period. Some women say that before this happens they stop feeling pregnant – symptoms such as fuller or tender breasts or nausea may fade. This spotting may go on for several days, and may cease – in which case the pregnancy will continue as normal – or it may progress, become heavier, and there may be period-like pains or severe cramping. If a woman has some bleeding this is known as a threatened miscarriage or threatened abortion (medical terminology does not distinguish between an induced abortion and a miscarriage, which can distress women who overhear doctors using the word 'abortion' in a much wanted pregnancy). If a miscarriage threatens there is about a 50–50 chance of losing the pregnancy. If the bleeding becomes very severe or if there is a lot of pain, this is usually an inevitable abortion – either the foetus is dead or the cervix (entrance to the womb) is open and nothing can save the pregnancy.

When a miscarriage occurs after the first three months of pregnancy, it may follow a similar pattern or it may be very sudden, without the warning bleeding and without much pain.

A miscarriage may be comparatively quick and painless or it may involve a long labour. Some doctors may give painkilling injections or even an epidural as in childbirth, but this is rare. Once the miscarriage is over the woman usually is given a D and C (dilatation and curettage, or scraping of the womb) to make sure that nothing is left behind which could lead to an infection or haemorrhage, or damage the woman's future fertility.

What causes a miscarriage?

In the majority of cases the cause of any individual miscarriage is never found. Miscarriages are so common that doctors will not investigate unless there are some particular special circumstances, or unless the woman has had three miscarriages or more. In most cases the woman conceives again before too long and has a normal pregnancy.

If a woman does have several miscarriages, however, doctors will usually investigate. If the miscarriages occur at different times in pregnancy, this is normally referred to as recurrent abortion and is usually the result of extreme bad

luck. If the miscarriages occur at the same time in pregnancy and with the same symptoms, this is known as
habitual abortion and is usually traced to the same medical
cause.

Most miscarriages seem to be caused by once-only accidents in the whole complex process of pregnancy. The
processes of fertilisation, early growth of the embryo,
implantation of the fertilised egg into the lining of the
womb and the establishment of the right environment for
the foetus to develop are all very complex and delicate,
and it is not surprising that sometimes things go wrong.

'Blighted ovum'

Women who miscarry sometimes hear the term 'blighted
egg' or 'blighted ovum' used to explain what went wrong.
This means that either the egg or the sperm which fertilised
it were abnormal, and so the fertilised egg failed to develop.
This will usually result in early miscarriage. Some women
who have also had normal pregnancies say that often in
such a pregnancy they do not 'feel pregnant' even though a
pregnancy test is positive.

Hormonal problems

Another reason for miscarriage may be hormonal problems. This is actually much rarer than was once thought, as
nowadays doctors tend to think that a decrease in levels of
progesterone, a hormone necessary to sustain a pregnancy,
is a symptom and not a cause of failed pregnancy. Some
women may have a progesterone deficiency which is not
enough to prevent pregnancy but severe enough to allow a
miscarriage to occur. This can usually be established by
taking blood samples and screening these for the level of
hormone throughout a woman's monthly cycle.

Some women seem to produce too high a level of the hormone testosterone, usually thought of as a male hormone but also produced in smaller quantities in women. Illnesses such as over- or under-functioning of the thyroid or adrenal glands, or diabetes, can also affect a pregnancy. Acute illness with high fever such as severe influenza or some rare viral infections can occasionally affect a pregnancy.

Many miscarriages do seem to occur around the 12-week mark. This is a very delicate time in a pregnancy, when the womb suddenly starts to expand rapidly as the foetus begins to grow apace, and when the task of maintaining hormone levels switches from the corpus luteum – the follicle in the ovary from which the egg was released – to the placenta itself. In some cases the fall in hormone levels may come too soon and the pregnancy will fail.

In some cases abnormalities of the womb – the presence of fibroids (see page 32) or an abnormal womb with an extra partition or septum, or a double (bicornuate) womb may cause miscarriages.

'Incompetent' cervix

After 13 weeks, miscarriages are either caused by problems in the attachment of the placenta to the wall of the uterus, or by what is known as an 'incompetent cervix'. The muscles around the entrance to the womb are very strong, and need to be so if they are to hold the growing weight of the foetus and the sac of water enclosing it. If the cervix is weak – usually after having been stretched too much in an earlier pregnancy, or during an induced abortion or an operation such as a D and C – the cervix may dilate too soon in the pregnancy and cause the bag of waters and the foetus to be expelled.

Moles
An occasional abnormality of pregnancy which can cause miscarriage is a hydatidiform mole, which occurs in about one in 2,000 pregnancies, but is more common in older women. In a molar pregnancy a great deal of placental tissue is formed, but no embryo. The woman often feels sick due to overproduction of placental hormones and the pregnancy may seem too large for the dates. Usually the mole is miscarried, or it may be picked up by an ultrasound scan.

Immunological problems
Some women have repeated miscarriages, sometimes very early on in the pregnancy, and seem unable to carry a baby to term. Often this is because the woman or her partner is carrying a chromosomal abnormality which means that these babies would be abnormal. It has recently been recognised that some women miscarry because they are rejecting the baby in their womb as a foreign body and expel it. There is a very complicated mechanism which prevents the immune system from rejecting the baby and allows the mother's body to tolerate a 'foreign body' in her womb; in some couples who have similar tissue types this process fails to work properly. Professors Beard and Mowbray at St Mary's Hospital, Paddington, found that immunising the mother with an injection of her partner's white blood cells can overcome this rejection problem and enable her to have a normal pregnancy.

Preventing miscarriages

Unfortunately there has been little progress in understanding what can be done to prevent miscarriages. Because a high proportion of miscarried foetuses are abnormal, doctors do not want to intervene and prolong a pregnancy where the foetus cannot survive or will be born abnormal.

If the cause is an abnormality of the womb, such as fibroids or a septum, surgery can help. If an incompetent cervix is diagnosed, a doctor can stitch the muscles of the cervix at around 14 weeks before a miscarriage can occur, and then remove these a week or two before the baby is due in a simple procedure.

With most miscarriages, the usual treatment suggested is bed rest. Some doctors recommend that the woman lies down all the time, only getting up to go to the toilet; others that she should simply take things very easy. There is a medical reason why this is advised; if the placenta is becoming detached, rest may help to allow it to become attached more firmly again. But usually it is thought that rest 'can't do any harm' and it is a way of relieving a woman's anxiety by making her feel she is doing everything she can to save the pregnancy. Most women threatening to miscarry instinctively want to rest. However, one study comparing women who rested with another group who couldn't – usually those with other small children to look after – found there was no difference in outcome in the two groups.

This study contradicts other evidence, however. One large study of women who had both planned and unplanned pregnancies showed that while 12 per cent of women with planned, wanted pregnancies had miscarriages, those who had conceived accidentally – all of whom were still using a method of contraception – had twice as many miscarriages. This does not count women who had IUDs, as the rate of miscarriage in women who conceive with an IUD in place is very high – about 60 per cent.

The man who conducted this study, Professor Martin Vessey, says that these results are 'highly significant' but no further research has been done as to why more of the unwanted pregnancies failed. There was no question of women trying to interfere with the pregnancy, as all were offered an early, safe legal abortion. However, Professor Vessey suggests that the women who conceived by accident may have been less 'careful' with the pregnancy – perhaps smoking and drinking more, playing strenuous sports, or generally 'neglecting' the pregnancy.

The best advice to be given, especially if you have had more than one miscarriage, is to avoid drinking alcohol and smoking, travel or strenuous activity, or stressful situations. It may also be suggested that you don't have sexual intercourse until after the time that your previous miscarriage occurred if you are worried about this triggering another miscarriage.

Receiving sympathy and support in a subsequent pregnancy can also help reduce the chance of miscarriage. One study carried out by a GP showed that women who were given support and reassurance during their next pregnancies were less likely to have a miscarriage than other women. This shows that psychological factors may be at work, and that it is important that women who miscarry should be given information, comfort and reassurance.

Coping with a miscarriage

A miscarriage is a very distressing experience; apart from the physical trauma, you have lost the life which was growing inside you. It can be particularly distressing if you have waited a long time to conceive or if this is a very late baby and you feel you may be running out of time. A miscarriage is a real bereavement and you should not expect to get over it quickly. It is normally recommended that you wait three months before trying to conceive again, as a pregnancy that occurs very soon after a miscarriage may be more likely to fail again. Women are sometimes advised to wait longer to give themselves time to recover mentally, but many older women will want to get on with another pregnancy as quickly as possible, especially if they are in their late thirties or forties. You are bound to be a little nervous in a pregnancy which follows a miscarriage, but think positive; the chances are that you will go on to have a healthy baby in the end.

4

Antenatal screening

The majority of mothers over the age of 35 who become pregnant can hope to have a normal pregnancy and a healthy baby. However, there are higher risks of the mother developing complications, therefore she needs to be screened to detect these at an early stage. Older mothers are also at higher risk of having an abnormal baby, so most are keen to take advantage of the screening tests that are available.

There can hardly be a mother who has not worried at some time in her pregnancy whether her baby will be normal, and this may be particularly true for the older mother. Fortunately, there are now a number of screening tests offered to women who are at higher risk of having an abnormal baby. These tests can be very important in setting the parents' minds at rest or, in cases where an abnormality is shown, in enabling them to decide whether or not to proceed with a pregnancy. However, it is important to remember that not all abnormalities can be detected in pregnancy and that accidents at birth can also lead to handicap. The tests eliminate certain problems but do not guarantee the 'perfect baby'.

How the baby develops

A human embryo is more or less completely formed by the end of the twelfth week of pregnancy. After this time it simply has to grow in size and its organs have to mature to make it capable of living outside the womb. All the major developments take place in the early weeks of pregnancy, which is why it is most important to look after yourself before you even know you are pregnant. The baby's spinal column, for example, is beginning to form in the fifth week of pregnancy. You are likely at this stage to realise that your period is late, but have not had a pregnancy confirmed. In the sixth week arm and leg buds are formed and in the seventh week the beginnings of the fingers and toes are visible and dramatic changes are occurring to the head and face. In the ninth week the nose and mouth take shape and by the eleventh week the genitals are formed, and all the internal organs are functioning.

Abnormalities in a baby are usually caused by genetic problems or by an environmental influence, such as poor diet, the use of drugs in early pregnancy or by hazards in the workplace, such as toxic chemicals or radiation. Genetic problems fall into two categories: those which are caused by either or both parents carrying a faulty gene, or those which occur when the sperm or egg are formed and involve an extra chromosome or part of a chromosome being included in the fertilised egg.

Chromosomes are the essential components of every living cell which determine not only how each cell works, but how the whole organism grows, develops, functions and looks. The chromosomes are made up of smaller units called genes, each of which determines a particular characteristic of the organism. Each different animal and plant species has its unique number and size of chromosomes, carrying all the relevant genes. In humans there are 46 chromosomes in 23 pairs. One set is inherited from the mother and one set from the father of each individual.

When the human cells divide to create the sperm or the egg, the pairs of chromosomes are mixed and separated at random so that each egg and each sperm carries a different set of genes, although there will always be one of each pair. This is why every human being is different. One of the pairs of chromosomes determines the baby's sex; these are called the X and Y chromosomes, because of their shape when viewed under the microscope. When sperm are formed, half will carry the Y chromosome which determines maleness, and half the X chromosome. All eggs carry the X chromosome. It is therefore the father who determines the sex of a baby.

Very occasionally the process of division will go wrong and the sperm or egg cell will end up with an extra chromosome, or sometimes an extra part of a chromosome, and when sperm and egg fuse the embryo will be faulty. In most cases these abnormal sperm, eggs or embryos will not be able to survive or, if the embryo does develop, the baby cannot survive long. It is thought that a high proportion – as many as 50 per cent – of miscarriages are caused by the embryo being abnormal.

Sometimes, however, the presence of an extra chromosome does not prevent the baby from developing or living. The most common of these instances is when there is an extra one of the twenty-first pair of chromosomes, which causes Down's syndrome. Other chromosomal abnormalities which are not lethal are when a girl lacks an X chromosome (Turner's syndrome) or a boy has an extra X (Klinefelter's syndrome) or an extra Y chromosome.

Apart from chromosomal abnormalities, other diseases and handicaps are caused by a faulty gene. Literally hundreds of inherited illnesses are now known, although most are extremely rare. Some of these are caused by a dominant gene, others – and these are more common – by a recessive gene.

A dominant gene is one which will always show itself if it is present, while a recessive gene can remain hidden, perhaps for generations. Each individual inherits one gene for each characteristic from each parent. Suppose the child inherits one gene for blue eyes and one gene for brown. Rather than the two colours being merged, what happens is that one gene is dominant over the other – brown eyes dominate blue, so the individual has brown eyes. However, he still carries a gene for blue eyes which, if it is paired with another gene for blue eyes in his future partner, can express itself in the next generation.

Two relatively well known, dominantly inherited diseases are Huntington's chorea, a degenerative nerve disease which does not show up till the third or fourth decade of life, and achondroplasia, a form of dwarfism which is linked to older fathers. If a person has a dominantly inherited disease, they have a 50 per cent chance of having an affected child.

Recessively inherited diseases are more insidious as they can be carried by large numbers of people without their knowledge. As long as the recessive gene is only paired with normal genes, there is no problem. However, if two people carrying the abnormal gene have children, there is a one-in-four chance of their baby having the disease; and other children are likely to be carriers.

Recessively inherited diseases include cystic fibrosis, Tay Sachs disease, sickle-cell anaemia, and phenylketonuria.

Some of these can be treated if diagnosed early (all babies in this country have a tiny pinprick of blood taken in the first week of life to test for diseases like phenylketonuria). Others can be tested for during pregnancy.

Many genes are carried in the X chromosomes and these cause sex-linked diseases if they are abnormal. If a person is female and has two X chromosomes, the abnormal gene is likely to be masked by a normal gene. If it is paired with a Y chromosome, however, there may be no normal gene to mask it as the Y chromosome is shorter and carries fewer genes. Examples of sex-linked diseases are haemophilia and Duchenne muscular dystrophy.

Some congenital abnormalities are caused not by a simple faulty gene but by a combination of factors. Perhaps several faulty genes are involved, or a combination of a faulty gene with some environmental stimulus, such as a drug taken in pregnancy, or an inadequate diet. Neural tube defects (anencephaly and spina bifida), cleft lip palate and some congenital heart defects are caused in this way. Indeed, there may be a random element, too. There have been recorded cases of identical twins being born where one had a cleft lip and the other did not.

Fortunately, most of these problems are relatively rare. But abnormalities such as Down's syndrome and spina bifida are more common and more likely to be a cause of concern. On the other hand, these are the abnormalities which can be detected by tests in the early stages of pregnancy.

Down's Syndrome

This is the most common chromosomal abnormality and affects about one in 600 live-born infants in Britain. The risk of having a Down's syndrome baby does increase with the mother's age. At the age of 20, a woman has nearly a one in 2,000 chance of having an affected child. At the age of 30 this has risen to about one in 900, and by 40 about one in 100. After this it rises still more steeply, so that a mother of 43 has a one in 50 chance and a mother of 47 a one in 20 chance. By the age of 50 the chance is about one in 10. (see Graph 4.1). There is also evidence that the risk of having a Down's syndrome baby increases if the father is over 55.

The most significant problem faced by Down's syndrome children is that they are mentally handicapped, although the degree of handicap varies; some can, with help and stimulation, achieve IQs of about 80, considered to be the dull end of the normal spectrum; many have IQs of less than 50 and are severely mentally handicapped. Down's syndrome children can also be recognised by their flattened profile, slanted eyes with an extra fold (hence the label Mongol) and stubby fingers. Most grow slowly and are small for their age, and many have additional handicaps – heart defects, eye abnormalities, hearing problems and a tendency to respiratory infections are common. Down's syndrome babies are characteristically 'floppy' at birth and many have problems with breast feeding as they may lack the strength to feed properly as well as the reflex to suck.

Most women expect to have a normal healthy baby when they go into labour, although a very small number may know that their baby is likely to be born handicapped. When things go wrong and a woman has to face up to this at the time of the birth, the shock and disbelief can be quite devastating.

'They told us after the birth that she wasn't normal. I refused to listen. I said, "If you're worried about her

Chromosome risks by maternal age at term delivery

Maternal age	Down's Syndrome risk	Chromosomal abnormalities risk
20–21	1/1,167	1/526
22–23	1/1,429	1/500
24–25	1/1,250	1/476
26	1/1,176	1/476
27	1/1,111	1/455
28	1/1,053	1/435
29	1/1,000	1/417
30	1/952	1/385
31	1/909	1/385
32	1/769	1/322
33	1/602	1/286
34	1/485	1/238
35	1/378	1/192
36	1/289	1/156
37	1/224	1/127
38	1/173	1/102
39	1/136	1/83
40	1/106	1/66
41	1/82	1/53
42	1/63	1/42
43	1/49	1/33
44	1/38	1/26
45	1/30	1/21
46	1/23	1/16
47	1/18	1/13
48	1/14	1/10
49	1/11	1/8

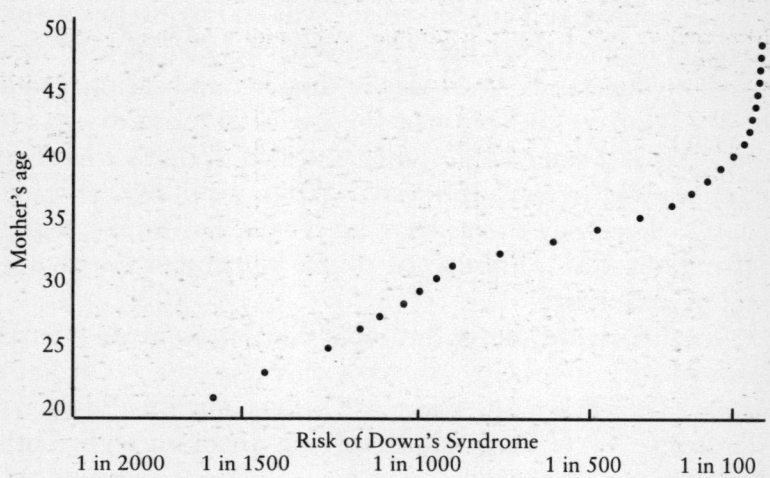

slanting eyes, my other children had that, they're my husband's eyes." Then they showed me how she didn't have the normal reflexes and how floppy she was and one or two other things, and I had to believe it was true. My husband was also told and he didn't know what to say; we couldn't look at one another. My first feeling for the baby was absolute hate: I hated her for not being normal. I seriously thought of having her adopted. That feeling lasted a day or two.'

It may take the parents days, weeks and sometimes even months to accept what has happened and to acknowledge that a baby born with some form of handicap needs just as much love and care as a normal baby.

'I wouldn't talk to the other mothers, or the staff, wouldn't see my family, and wouldn't see the baby. Then I thought, she can't be that bad, I'll just go and look at her.

She was asleep (the nurses had been feeding her). I just looked and looked at her and she was so tiny, so beautiful, like my other babies had been. I felt a rush of love and when my husband came I was feeding her and crying. I told him, "We have to keep her, she needs us more than anyone." He just smiled and smiled and said, "That's what I've been waiting to hear. It doesn't matter, we'll love her anyway." I won't say things have been easy, but I don't regret having her now, although of course sometimes I wish she had been normal.'

Down's syndrome is the most common chromosomal abnormality involving an extra chromosome – chromosome 21, in this case. There are others, such as Edward's syndrome, or trisomy 18, involving an extra eighteenth chromosome. Edward's syndrome is the most common trisomy after Down's syndrome, and occurs in about one in 5,000 live births. It leads to multiple congenital handicaps and most children die within a few days or weeks after birth, despite medical intervention. Edward's syndrome babies are usually small, with tiny features and pixie-like ears, and have internal heart and kidney abnormalities. As with other chromosomal abnormalities of this kind, there is some association with maternal age.

Neural tube defects

Neural tube defects, which include spina bifida and anencephaly, occur in about three in every 1,000 live births. There is no evidence that it is more common in older mothers. Early in pregnancy, a groove appears down the baby's back and this develops into the brain and spinal cord. Normally the groove closes into a tube in which the spinal cord and brain develop but in rare cases the tube does not close properly. If the defect is in the part of the tube that forms the brain, anencephaly results; this is always fatal as the upper skull and brain do not form. If the defect is lower down, then part of the spinal cord and nerves protrude, covered by a fragile membrane; the baby is usually paralysed from this point down. Sometimes, however, spina bifida can be less severe, is not visible from outside and results in minimal handicap.

As many as 85 per cent of babies severely affected with spina bifida also have a defect called hydrocephaly. Cerebro-spinal fluid accumulates in the head, causing mental retardation if untreated. Nowadays the fluid can be drained away after birth and surgery can repair the opening in the spine to reduce the risk of infection. Surgery and other techniques have improved the outlook for children suffering from this handicap.

Spina bifida can probably be largely prevented by an adequate diet before and during early pregnancy. Evidence has shown that taking vitamin supplements rich in B-group vitamins and folic acid has greatly reduced the incidence of spina bifida, even in mothers at greater risk because the handicap is in their family.

Cleft lip and palate

This is one of the most common abnormalities, affecting about one in 1,000 babies, and again, does not seem to be more common in older mothers. The cleft is caused when the tissues which move together to form the face in very early pregnancy do not fuse, leaving a gap which can involve the lip alone, the palate, or both. The cleft can be on one or both sides of the face and varies in its seriousness. The vast majority of children with cleft lip or palate are normal in other respects, but sometimes it is found accompanying some other abnormality.

Cleft palate can cause quite serious feeding problems in the early months, as the baby is unlikely to be able to suck well. The child will have difficulties in speaking and also teeth are likely to be missing or malformed in the area of the cleft. Plastic surgery, however, can now be carried out so that the cleft is completely repaired, inside and out, by the time the child reaches maturity. Speech therapy and orthodontic work are usually required.

Although cleft lip and palate are correctable, it is very distressing to give birth to an affected child:

'Our son was born with a double cleft palate and lip. When he was born it looked terribly disfiguring, because the middle of his upper lip and jaw were pushed forward, rather like a beak. He had terrible feeding problems; he couldn't suck, and had to be fed at first with a spoon. You can imagine how difficult this is with a hungry, crying baby whose every instinct is to suck. He had to have a series of operations throughout his childhood and the end result is very good. But the emotional effects of stays in hospital and of looking different to other children are harder to deal with than the physical repairs.'

Abnormalities in the digestive tract

Also relatively common and correctable defects, not normally related to maternal age, are abnormalities in the digestive tract. These include a blockage of the entrance to the stomach, often accompanied by an oesophageal/

tracheal fistula, where the windpipe and gullet are joined; and blockages at various points in the digestive tract, including an imperforate anus. All these are quite easily corrected by surgery and some can even be detected in the womb by ultrasound.

Detecting abnormalities

Some tests are now available to screen all mothers, and others are available for those mothers who are at higher risk of having a handicapped child. Some of these tests are offered to women routinely, others only to women over a certain age who are already known to be at risk either because of family history or because of previous difficulties with pregnancies. Most maternity hospitals will explain at the booking-in clinic what their procedure is and which tests they offer to women. If they don't, and you would like to know, ask which tests they offer and when they do them.

Screening tests include ultrasound scans, which are now performed routinely at 16 weeks at many hospitals; a blood test which can detect raised levels of a substance called alphafetoprotein in the blood which may indicate a neural tube defect; amniocentesis – taking a sample of the waters surrounding the baby which enables the chromosomes to be examined, showing up a chromosomal abnormality and, incidentally, showing the child's sex; and rarer techniques such as fetoscopy, where the baby can be examined through a tube inserted into the womb, and chorionic villi sampling, a new experimental technique which may one day replace amniocentesis.

Ultrasound

Since the 1970s, remarkable improvements in ultrasound technology have meant that it has opened up a real 'window on the womb'. Ultrasound consists of high frequency sound waves which are bounced off the baby to give a photographic picture of the foetus. Unlike X-rays, which have much higher powers of penetration, ultrasound will show up soft tissues and thus can give a complete picture of the growing baby, and is a very useful diagnostic tool.

An ultrasound scan tends to be given to all women at around 16 weeks of pregnancy in hospitals which have the equipment. If not, women who may be at special risk because of problems with a previous pregnancy, or who would like to have a scan, can often be referred to a hospital where it can be performed. The reasons given for the routine use of ultrasound is that the pregnancy can be very accurately dated at around 16 weeks by measuring the circumference of the baby's head, and this is very useful in avoiding problems later if the mother is unsure of her dates and does not know when the baby is due. The scan can also locate the position of the placenta, which can shed light on any bleeding later in pregnancy, and can be used to check that the baby has no major physical abnormalities such as anencephaly or stunted limbs. Ultrasound can also show up congenital heart defects, kidney disease and other severe abnormalities. Ultrasound can also detect if the mother is expecting more than one baby.

There has been some controversy about the safety of ultrasound, which has caused concern to women who are not sure whether they should accept a routine scan. Ultrasound has now been in use for many years without any evidence of harmful effects to the baby. Recently, the Royal College of Obstetricians and Gynaecologists issued a report recommending no change in the policy of carrying out routine scans at 16–18 weeks of pregnancy. In England and Wales 72 per cent of mothers have routine scans and a further 13 per cent have a scan for medical reasons, so some 85 per cent of mothers will have at least one scan in the course of their pregnancy.

All the indications are that the benefits of having ultrasound outweigh any potential risk. Not least is the benefit of reassurance given to many women on seeing their baby is alive and well, particularly those who have waited a long time to have a baby or who have experienced a miscarriage. However, a large study carried out in the States by the National Institutes of Health on 15,000 women with a low risk of problems in pregnancy showed that while the detection of twins and malformations was increased and pregnancy could be dated more accurately, the outcome – in terms of healthy babies – was not improved. There was no difference in the rate of foetal or neonatal death or subsequent illness. The rates of preterm birth, the outcomes of postdate pregnancies, and low birth weight babies were similar. Although the percentage of abnormal foetuses detected in the group who had ultrasound was three times higher, the abortion rate was about the same in both groups.

So, while ultrasound is of undoubted benefit in women at high risk or in special situations where a problem is detected, its routine benefits are yet unproved. The use of ultrasound can help some mothers anxious about their pregnancies through reassurance, but can also create anxieties for others:

'Towards the end of my pregnancy they started to worry

about whether my baby was growing properly. I don't know what started it all off, but once they'd got this idea into their heads they wouldn't leave me alone. I was in and out of hospital having blood pressure taken and having ultrasound scan after scan. My blood pressure was up – no doubt with all the worry – and they couldn't decide what to do. They said that they would have to induce the baby early to make sure that all would be well and then they changed their minds and decided to wait. I was in hospital for the last few weeks of the pregnancy and, of course, the baby decided to be late. They let me go two weeks overdue and then they decided induce the birth, and by then I was so desperate I said, "Yes." It was a terrible birth ending with an emergency Caesarean, and when he was born he was 7lb 1oz. Nor did he look overdue. I asked the consultant later, "So what happened about this small baby?" There was nothing wrong at all, my worries had been for nothing. They said they couldn't explain it but he had appeared small on the scan. So much for all their wonderful technology!'

Some women – and doctors and midwives, too – feel that, with the increased reliance on new technology, many of the old skills in obstetrics are being lost:

'I had shared care and I noticed a tremendous difference between my visits to the hospital and my visits to my very experienced GP. At the hospital people seemed to poke and probe for a long time and suggested that I might have another scan to check the baby was growing OK. When I went to my GP she examined me very quickly and said, "Oh, this baby's doing fine, I should think he weighs about 4lb now." I asked how she knew and she just said, "Experience." It seems that in hospitals you only see the young junior staff and the consultants are just called out for special occasions; no wonder you don't always get the best care and they give you all sorts of unnecessary tests.'

Having an ultrasound scan

An ultrasound scan is a simple, non-invasive procedure. In early pregnancy you are usually asked to drink a lot of water an hour or two before your appointment and not to empty your bladder. This pushes the womb up in the pelvis and will give the ultrasound operator a clearer view. You will be asked to lie down on a couch and remove any clothing that covers your abdomen. A cold jelly is then rubbed over the abdomen to enable the ultrasound operator to move the scanner smoothly over the area. As she does so you will see the baby's outline appear on the television screen and you will also see the foetal movements. It can be quite difficult to interpret what you are seeing so, if you are not told, do ask. The operator can freeze the picture at any moment and point things out to you at length without exposing the baby to any more sound waves than are necessary. You will usually be able to see the baby's head, the arms and legs moving around, and some of the internal organs at work. You may even be able to see the baby sucking his thumb:

'The woman took a lot of time to explain to me about what she was looking for and what she could see. I found all this terribly reassuring. She pointed out the heart beating, the cord and the placenta, the kidneys and the spine and showed me how much he was moving around.'

Other women find the process unnerving especially if nothing is explained.

'No one said anything to me and I was afraid to ask in case anything was wrong. She kept on looking at everything and taking measurements and I started to get very jumpy. Then she suddenly got up and said, "I just want to get a second opinion on this" and I was terrified. I thought, "This is it. Something's terribly wrong." I was in tears. Someone else came back and they were both looking at the screen, still not saying anything to me. "What is it, what is wrong?" I finally asked. "Nothing's wrong, I'm just checking these measurements." I felt as if I wasn't a person, a mother, just a scientific toy.'

Usually the baby's father is welcome to come and watch the process and see the baby on the screen. Many find this a very positive experience, as they are able to give support, but also the baby becomes real to them in an even more dramatic way than to the woman: 'It was hard for me to take in that she was pregnant until I saw the baby on the screen. It was fantastic – it made it come alive for me.'

Increasingly ultrasound is being used to detect a range of abnormalities. It may now be possible to use it to detect Down's syndrome and other chromosomal abnormalities. One new development is the Nuchal Translucency Scan, developed at the Harris Birthright Research Centre for Foetal Medicine and King's College Hospital, London, and is still part of a research project. During an ultrasound scan which can be carried out as early as 11 weeks' gestation, doctors measure the 'black space' behind the neck of the foetus. A large space of 3mm or more may indicate the presence of a nuchal membrane associated with abnormality.

Alphafetoprotein blood test

This test is a routine blood test carried out at between 16 and 18 weeks of pregnancy. It measures the level of a substance called alphafetoprotein (AFP) which gets into the mother's bloodstream from the baby. A high level of alphafetoprotein can mean a number of things: that the pregnancy is further advanced than was thought, that the mother is expecting twins, or that the baby is suffering from a neural tube defect. It can also mean nothing at all!

If a woman does have a higher than normal level of AFP, a second blood test will be done to confirm this. If this too is positive, then there is a roughly one-in-seven chance that the foetus has a neural tube defect. It is usually recommended that the woman have an ultrasound scan to check for the presence of anencephaly or spina bifida. If all this is inconclusive, an amniocentesis is usually recommended so that the level of AFP in the amniotic fluid can be measured (see section below).

The problem with the AFP blood test is that for every ten women with a raised AFP level, only one will have a cause found. The other nine will have a normal baby, although they may have a slightly greater risk of having a small for dates baby. The majority of women with a high AFP level will have a 'positive' result, and then an amniocentesis performed, accompanied by all the stress and worry involved, when there is actually nothing wrong with their baby. The chance of the level of AFP being high from other causes is greater than the risk of there being a neural tube defect.

Rather than performing the AFP test routinely without the mother being fully consulted, it might be better to explain what the test is for and what it entails and let the mother choose. Some people will welcome it, others prefer to do without:

'I had just had the scan, seen the baby moving, that its head was there and it was kicking its legs. I thought, we would have seen if there was anything really wrong, its head would have been the wrong shape or its legs paralysed.

Anyway, I felt I couldn't possibly have aborted that baby once I had seen him like that. So I decided not to have the test. What was the point of having it done when I could see there was nothing so very wrong with the baby and wouldn't have wanted an abortion anyway?'

Further, not all neural tube defects are detected by the test. There is no absolute level of AFP in the amniotic fluid at which one can say, this baby is affected and this one isn't, an artificial line has to be drawn. If the level is set too high, more neural tube defects will be undetected. If it is too low, more women will have further tests with all the worry attached or even have an abortion when there is nothing wrong with their baby.

A new test known as the Triple Test has been developed at Bart's hospital and is now offered to mothers in about two-thirds of health authorities. A blood test is taken at 16 weeks and levels of alphafetoprotein are measured, together with two other 'markers', unconjugated oestriol and human chorionic gonadotrophin (HCG). High levels of AFP may mean spina bifida, while low levels of AFP and unconjugated oestradiol together with high levels of HCG indicate a higher risk of having a Down's syndrome baby.

The results are combined with the woman's age to give her a 'risk factor'. A risk of one in 250 or higher is considered 'screen positive' – i.e., an amniocentesis or further screening is advised. A risk of less than one in 250 is considered 'screen negative'. However, a positive result means, on average, only a 1 in 50 chance of the woman having a Down's syndrome baby. Again, there is concern that too many women will be put under great stress by receiving a 'positive' test result and having an amniocentesis.

There is another development of this test, the Triple Plus, where another marker – neutrophil alkaline phosphatase –

is measured in a costly process. This makes the test more accurate, but at the time of writing it is only available privately because of the cost.

Amniocentesis

Amniocentesis (testing the waters) consists of taking a sample of the amniotic fluid surrounding the baby and analysing it. The amniotic fluid contains some of the baby's cells, and these can be cultured to show up any chromosomal abnormalities. Amniocentesis can also be used to detect neural tube defects, as there will then be a very high level of AFP in the amniotic fluid; this is much more accurate than the AFP blood test.

Amniocentesis is usually offered to women over the age of 37 or 38 although policies differ from hospital to hospital and region to region. A survey carried out by the Maternity Alliance some years ago showed that this test would be available to three-quarters of women over the age of 38. Most NHS doctors are reluctant to carry out the test before the age of 35, because there is only a one in 300 chance of finding an abnormality at this age, while the chance of causing a miscarriage is about one in 150. By the age of 40, on the other hand, the chance of an abnormality has risen to more than one in 100. If a consultant is unwilling to carry out the test despite a couple's worries, they can try asking a consultant who is more sympathetic to their viewpoint or, as a last resort, have it done privately.

The risk of miscarriage attached to amniocentesis is small. Studies used to quote a rate of about 0.5–1 per cent, but one large scale study in Glasgow showed that the risk may be lower. They found a risk of only 0.7 per cent, 0.2

per cent if only miscarriages which occurred within two weeks of the procedure were counted. Some doctors dispute whether there is a real risk at all.

However, for older mothers, especially those with a history of miscarriage or infertility and for whom a pregnancy is particularly precious, there is a real fear of inducing a miscarriage and this can make the decision to have an amniocentesis a very difficult one.

Rita was unlucky and had a miscarriage a week after her amniocentesis at the age of 39. 'I was completely, utterly devastated. I blamed myself. They had told me the risk but it had seemed so small; I'd never heard of anyone actually losing a baby. They said it might not have been the amnio, that it might have happened anyway, but that seemed to me to be the most likely reason, because there was nothing wrong with the baby. It was a girl, and I had wanted a girl. I felt I had gone against nature and been punished. It was a terrible, terrible time for me.

'I did get pregnant again a year later and I had a boy. I decided against an amnio and he is fine. Everything is fine, but now I'm 41 and I may not get pregnant again, and if I do, I now don't know whether to have an amnio or not. I keep thinking that if I hadn't had one I could now have had two children and my family would be complete. On the other hand, perhaps I should just count myself lucky that I am now a mother and have a healthy child.'

An amniocentesis is usually carried out at about 16 weeks into pregnancy. This is the earliest time that sufficient amniotic fluid can be drawn off for testing. Amniocentesis is done on an out-patient basis, so you will not have to be admitted to hospital. Amniocentesis is almost always done now at the same time as an ultrasound scan. This is done first to establish that you are at least 16 weeks pregnant and to see the exact position of the foetus and placenta. You are normally asked to have a full bladder for the scan and then to empty it before the amniocentesis is performed.

The needle is usually inserted without local anaesthetic, as the local anaesthetic really only means you get two pin-pricks instead of one. The doctor directs the needle into the amniotic fluid and draws off about 30 ml of the pale-yellow fluid. When ultrasound is used as well, the danger of the needle hitting the baby or placenta is very small. Most women do not find the procedure painful, and describe a slight cramp or pressure in the womb as the needle passes through the uterine wall. Some women feel a little sore for a day or two afterwards and you are usually advised to take it easy because of the slight risk of miscarriage. For some women, however, the test is not so straightforward:

'We went along at 16–17 weeks; my husband came and we were all keyed up. They did the scan first and said the baby was lying all spread out and there were no big pock-ets of fluid to get the needle into, so it wasn't worth trying. We had to go back the following week – the anticlimax was awful.'

'While pregnant with Max at the age of 35 I did worry a lot that he might be handicapped. I was feeling very aware of my age. When I was pregnant with Douglas at 37 I said that I did want an amnio. I was told that the risk of this causing a miscarriage was about the same as the risk of the baby having Down's syndrome and that I should only con-sider the test if I was prepared to have an abortion.

'I did feel that I couldn't handle having a handicapped child, and that it wouldn't be fair on the two boys. I had babysat for a mentally handicapped child and had no illu-sions about how difficult it was and how it had affected her brother. I would certainly have had a termination if anything had been wrong.

'They made light of the procedure, said I didn't need someone with me, it wouldn't take long, and that it wouldn't hurt. I was 16 weeks pregnant. Alan drove me to the hospital and waited outside. I was not given an anaesthetic. Ultrasound was used to locate the baby and the bag of fluid. An enormous-looking needle was stuck into my very tender belly and it was excruciatingly painful. I gripped the nurse's hand and counted to 60; the nurse kept saying, "It doesn't usually hurt." Then it was all over. I was shaking and very distressed. Alan had to help me to the car; there is no way I could have got home by myself. I started having contractions when I got home and these lasted for four hours, but I didn't bleed. I thought, oh God, what have I done? I'm going to lose the baby. I had to stay in bed all day and took things easy the next day.

'Waiting was OK for the first three weeks. Then the results were late, over four weeks, so I thought something must be wrong and started to get very depressed. Although they said they would only tell the mother the results I couldn't face ringing and got Alan to phone from the office. They told him all was well and we were both thrilled, though my mother burst into tears when I told her it was another boy. Horrible though the whole thing was, it was better than another four months of worrying and I felt I could look forward happily to the baby.'

Others find the process much easier than they thought:

'It was very simple. I felt absolutely nothing. My husband was there and he said "Did you really not feel anything because they seemed to take pints of fluid!" They were extremely helpful and reassuring and it was much, much easier than I had imagined it would be.'

Once the test is done the fluid has to be sent off to be analysed. The cells in the fluid have to be cultured and grown over a couple of weeks, then crushed and looked at under a microscope so the chromosomes can be examined. Very occasionally the test fails and has to be repeated, two or three weeks further into the pregnancy:

'I had an amnio at 16 weeks after much thought and consultation. The first one didn't take – and I had another at 20 weeks by which time I had felt the baby moving I couldn't understand what was wrong with the first test and worried that it meant that something was wrong with the baby.'

The fluid is also tested for high levels of alphafetoprotein which indicates the presence of a neural tube defect.

If you are the possible carrier of a genetic disease then tests can be carried out to identify up to 70 or 80 hereditary diseases. These tests are very time-consuming and expensive, so they will only be done if there is a history of an inherited illness which can be tested for in your family.

Waiting for the results can be the most difficult aspect of the whole procedure. Usually, women are told that the results will take three weeks, though sometimes it is sooner and rarely later: 'They said the results would take three weeks but in fact it was only two. They had tried to ring but we were out so they wrote us a very nice letter saying all was well.'

You are usually informed by letter or by telephone; you can telephone if the results are overdue. You can also ask to know the sex of the baby if you want to, though some hospitals insist on talking this over with you first:

'We had asked to know the sex of the baby but they were actually quite reluctant that we should know. They said go home and think about it, and asked probing questions about did we want a girl or boy. When they rang up to say the results were fine they didn't volunteer the information but we pressed it and they said it was a girl. We didn't really mind the sex, but we both had a slight preference for a girl. We were delighted and it was wonderful to know, which I hadn't in my earlier pregnancies. In fact, knowing was one of the most important parts of the pregnancy.'

There is some evidence that people who desperately want either a son or daughter have problems adjusting to the baby if they know in advance that it is the 'wrong' sex. In the heat of the birth itself, most parents are so pleased to know the baby is all right that they do not mind so much about its sex and the baby is there to love and care for. Knowing while pregnant, however, gives a parent time to brood over the as yet unknown person and sometimes to reject the baby, making it more difficult to adjust when the baby arrives.

This is a very individual matter and people hold very different attitudes:

'Of course I wanted to know. I thought if it was there in my notes and other people knew, then of course I had the right to know.'

'I told them, don't tell me! I didn't want to know, it would have spoiled it all, like unwrapping a present before your birthday.'

'If it's a first baby, I think once you know you feel rather sad in any case, because you want both, you can't really decide which is your preference. So when they said it's a girl, I felt sad in a way that it wasn't a boy though it wasn't that I actually wanted a boy.'

Most hospitals will respect people's wishes in the matter although some will provide limited counselling to help a couple decide whether they want to know or not. Occasionally one partner wants to know the sex and the other doesn't; this is very hard to deal with. If one partner is told and hides it from the other, it casts a considerable strain over a relationship at a time when a couple should be as close and open with one another as possible.

Fetoscopy

This technique involves passing a very small tube containing a light and a lens into the womb so that the developing baby can be seen. The tube is introduced through a small incision made just above the pubic bone under a local anaesthetic. Fetoscopy is carried out in the second three months of pregnancy and samples of the baby's blood, skin and liver can be taken. A number of abnormalities can be detected by fetoscopy that could not be found out any other way, and it has recently been used to 'operate' on the unborn baby, allowing drugs and transfusions to be given directly into the baby's bloodstream.

The baby is usually viewed at around 16 weeks and blood samples taken between 17 and 22 weeks. External defects, to the face or limbs, and neural tube defects are clearly visible. Haemophilia and other blood disorders can be detected, as can some diseases of the metabolism. The technique is not used lightly, however, as there is a substantially increased risk of miscarriage, death of the baby in the womb or premature labour.

Chorionic villi sampling (CVS)

This is a relatively new technique which is now being offered in various hospitals as an alternative to amniocentesis. The great advantage of the test is that it can be carried out much earlier than amniocentesis, at around 10–12 weeks. Originally it was offered earlier, as early as 8 or 9 weeks, but this was suspended after evidence that CVS in the first nine weeks of pregnancy was associated with foetal limb defects. CVS gives the mother who finds that her baby is abnormal the chance of an earlier abortion which can be carried out simply, rather than induced labour after she has felt the baby moving.

The CVS test is carried out by passing a thin tube through the cervix (neck of the womb) and removing a tiny fragment of tissue from the placenta. This can be done without an anaesthetic and, as with amniocentesis, ultrasound is used to show the exact position of the foetus and placenta. The vagina is cleaned with some antiseptic solution beforehand to prevent germs being introduced into the womb.

The test is not painful, but it is uncomfortable for many women, rather like having a cervical smear taken or, some women say, like having an IUD (contraceptive coil) fitted. The test takes about 10–20 minutes and you will be able to go home after about one hour. As with amniocentesis, you may be advised to take things easy for a day or two because of the risk of miscarriage. At the moment, this risk seems to be about 1-in-50, two or three times more likely than with amniocentesis. It is hard to be sure at present, however, when the test has not been in use for long and when there are not many doctors trained and skilled in performing it.

CVS detects any chromosomal abnormalities as does

amniocentesis, but it will not show up neural tube defects. Women who have this test will therefore also be given the AFP blood test to detect spina bifida. The results can be available quite quickly, sometimes in a matter of days.

When an abnormality is found

The vast majority of women who have these screening tests in pregnancy are reassured that all is well, and this enables them, and older mothers in particular, to relax and enjoy the rest of their pregnancy. However, it is important to remember that not all problems can be detected and that the tests are not always foolproof, and that problems can occur at birth which can handicap a child.

In the small number of cases where an abnormality is found, however, the pregnancy is transformed from a happy event into a nightmare. Some women feel this is just as traumatic as losing a full-term baby, and the experience of knowing you are carrying a handicapped child and deciding whether or not to have a termination is one of the most difficult choices anyone can have to face. Often, too, hospitals are lacking in adequate support services and do not know how to deal with a couple's distress and grief. There is an organisation, Support After Termination for Abnormality (SATFA) which can help (see Useful Addresses).

Doctors may fail to explain the news well, or there may be confusion over the results:

'They rang and said that the baby was a girl and that there was a problem. She mentioned Down's syndrome and my mind went into a complete spin. She gave me an appointment to see the doctor and I went around in a complete daze; I couldn't bring myself to tell anyone. When I saw the consultant she explained that while my daughter would not suffer from Down's syndrome herself, one chromosome was abnormal, so any children she had would suffer from Down's syndrome. In other words, the baby I had for days been considering aborting would be perfectly normal.'

Another mother felt that the way the news was broken to her was far from satisfactory:

'They didn't ring up with the results of the amnio so in the end I rang them. They said, "Oh, yes, we can't discuss this over the phone, you must make an appointment to come in." I knew then that something was wrong, so I asked, "What is it? Is it Down's syndrome?" She said no, it wasn't, and I would have to wait till I saw the doctor. So we had to wait for the next day. They told us there was a high level of alphafetoprotein in the fluid and that it was likely the baby had spina bifida, and so they would like to do another scan to check as they hadn't picked it up before. This time they did. They all looked at the screen, not me, though there were tears pouring down my face all the time. The consultant explained what the outlook was and painted this dismal picture for the child. We decided on an abortion straight away, but for some bureaucratic reason had to wait. In the meantime I was given no support.'

A study carried out in the States by the National Institutes for Child Health showed that of parents who discover their baby is abnormal, 95 per cent decide on a termination. The figure is probably about the same in Britain. Some hospitals advise that if a couple know they do not want to have a termination they should not have the tests, to spare them 'unnecessary' expense. However, not all couples know till the decision is upon them and others feel they have the right to know in any case so that they can prepare themselves – both in a practical sense and from the emotional point of view:

'I was 40 and had had years of infertility problems, in fact had been told I would never conceive a couple of months before I did. We discussed the possibility of a handicapped child and decided to have an amnio, because we didn't want to cope with a handicapped baby. Before we had the scan we had decided on a termination if anything was wrong but when we actually saw the baby, we both came out and said, "This is it, we won't have a termination." But we still went ahead and had the amnio.'

'We would never have had a termination; I don't believe it's right. But if it had been a Down's syndrome or something, I would have wanted to know so we could prepare ourselves, read up about it, tell the family in advance. I don't see why they should keep that from you.'

It is a particularly harrowing experience if the mother is carrying a sex-linked genetic disease which affects only boys, such as haemophilia or Duchenne muscular dystrophy. The latter is a particularly distressing disease in which a child who appears normal at birth suffers a gradual loss of muscular strength, becomes progressively paralysed and finally dies at the age of about 20.

If the mother is known to be carrying the disease, there is a 50 per cent chance that a boy will have the disease. Amniocentesis can tell the parents the child's sex, but not whether he has the disease, so parents can be faced with the agonising choice of terminating the pregnancy if they are carrying a boy without knowing if he would be affected or not. A girl will stand a 50 per cent chance of being a carrier, but will not have the disease.

IVF has opened up a new possibility for people carrying

genetic diseases with pre-implantation diagnosis. Here the woman's ovaries would be stimulated to produce several eggs which are collected and fertilised '*in vitro*'. About three days after fertilisation one cell can be removed from each embryo and tested for presence of the faulty gene. Only the normal embryos would be reimplanted and the woman would have the hope of a pregnancy in which she didn't have to worry about carrying an affected child. However, she would have to go through the full IVF procedure. So far about 10 pregnancies have been achieved world-wide following pre-implantation diagnosis, the majority conceived at the Hammersmith Hospital, London, the only UK centre licensed to carry out this procedure.

Problems with screening

The existence of these tests does mean many women enjoy their pregnancy free of certain worries but it also presents some very difficult choices. Some women feel they can only embark on a pregnancy in later life because they have the option of discovering if the baby has chromosomal abnormality, while others feel uncertain:

'We agreed we couldn't have coped with a severely handicapped baby and had all the tests. But I don't think the tests being available influenced my decision to have a baby. Having a baby is a very emotional decision. I was glad to have the tests but I didn't really think about it in advance – I would have taken the risk.'

Other mothers regret the existence of such tests, as they feel it puts an extra strain on the pregnancy:

'As I was 38 when my first baby was conceived, I decided I would have the amniocentesis done. In fact, this turned the first six months of my pregnancy, a time which should have been a happy one for me, into a nightmare.

'First I refused to "bond" with the baby in my mind, in case there was something wrong with him or her. By the time the test was to be done, I had worked myself into quite a state about it, and convinced myself that the result would be a bad one.

'When the test was done I felt contractions as if I was starting labour which terrified me; later I had a threatened miscarriage, which I'm sure was connected. I heard sooner than I expected, but it was neither a positive nor a negative result, as the test hadn't taken. They said there was just time to repeat the test if I wanted, and after a great deal of agonising I decided to do this.

'Again I had to wait two weeks – in fact a little more – before the result came. All was clear, and I felt a great relief. But the whole business made me feel enormously protective towards my baby, not wanting him to be interfered with and, at the same time, alienated all that time from him in case he was abnormal.'

Because amniocentesis are normally carried out at 16–18 weeks, and the results take two to four weeks to come back, a woman can be as much as 22 weeks pregnant when she knows that her baby is abnormal. Recently it has been performed as early as 11½ weeks, allowing for vaginal abortion at 14 weeks. This means that she will have felt the baby move and that she will be having an abortion almost at the time when the baby could live if it were born prematurely. The abortion will be a proper labour, although the foetus is killed first by the injection of hypo-saline solution or chemicals into the womb. Labour is induced medically, usually with prostoglandins, and may well last a long time. Many women find the experience of labour without the reward at the end a terrible experience:

'I couldn't bear to think about it or talk about it. It was a travesty of everything I'd ever read about the glory and wonder of childbirth. It was agony, and I just wanted to be doped until it was all over. I wouldn't let my husband be there; I couldn't have borne it for him to have to suffer it too.'

Although choosing to have a termination is a terrible and shocking experience, those couples who do so find this preferable to bringing a severely handicapped child into the world. However, there are couples who do choose to bring up their handicapped children, or adopt other people's, and find great rewards in doing so:

'Of course we found it hard at first having a Down's baby, and we've had hard times since he was born, but in the end we just loved him – he's our child and he's brought a lot of love into our lives.'

Some mothers feel that the screening tests put too much pressure on them and medicalise the pregnancy. 'After my first baby was born at 37 I had all these tests and I felt I had been taken over by the doctors, spending hours at the hospital waiting. They were offering a whole variety of new tests, including a blood test which was supposed to detect a higher risk of Down's syndrome baby.

'After the blood test I got a phone call to say the result was positive. I was so distressed I couldn't understand what they were saying at first. They explained that the result was borderline but that I should come in and talk about an amniocentesis. They told me that the risk based on my age alone was 1-in-287 while with this test it was 1-in-100.

'Did he advise an amniocentesis? It was borderline. He thought it would put my mind at rest. I pointed out that until I'd had this blood test my mind was at rest. My husband and I talked it over and we decided to have the amnio. I hated it, I hated waiting for the results, which were fine. With the second baby 18 months later I opted out. Everybody said, but you're at more risk, but I just didn't want to know. I turned down everything, even the AFP blood test. My GP was supportive about it; he said it was my right. The pregnancy and birth were very straightforward and I had a very healthy child.'

5

The birth – natural or not?

The last decade has seen considerable changes in how child-birth is seen by doctors, with guidelines from the Department of Health now admitting that mothers should be able to choose their position during labour, and delivery and giving much higher profile to the mother's wishes. Hospitals may now offer birthing stools, water pools, and other 'natural childbirth' props. Home births may be marginally more common and well accepted than they were a decade ago.

However, despite this progress, many women are still concerned that there is too much medical intervention in the process of childbirth. This is especially true for older mothers, who are seen to be at higher risk and are much more likely to receive medical intervention.

Home births are still very rare – planned home deliveries account for less than 1 per cent of the total – and few doctors would be happy about a first-time mother over 35 giving birth at home. Of course, the ultimate decision is yours, and you still have the option of a home birth if you want one, perhaps with the help of an independent mid-wife.

Denise had her first baby at home at the age of 42. 'I was in Germany when I got pregnant and they said I would have a planned Caesarean. I accepted this, but when I came to England when I was seven months pregnant I wanted a birth where I could have some continuity of care, as I had had in Germany. At an active birth class which I enrolled in I heard about independent midwives and decided this was what I wanted. Nobody mentioned a Caesarean.

'I did say I wanted to go into hospital – right up to the end I thought this. But I had read a lot about natural birth and I was interested. I suppose subconsciously I must have made up my mind, because when I went into labour, a week early, and the midwife came, she said at a certain point that if I was going into hospital I should go now, and I said, "No".

'I think being older gave me more confidence . . . I don't get overawed or intimidated by doctors. But I wouldn't have done it without the independent midwife's support . . . She was so confident, and I had absolute faith in her. It had been a normal pregnancy and the labour was progressing normally, so there seemed no reason to think anything would go wrong. I am sure that if I'd been in hospital there would have been intervention – I did find it incredibly more painful than I imagined, and I was yelling the place down. I think its very important to have someone with you who knows you, so that they can tell if you really need something or not.

'Afterwards I received a lot of criticism from people – that I could have put my child in danger, that I must have been incredibly brave, and so on. I found that very hard to cope with because I really didn't feel this was the case.'

Any first time mother over 40 is likely to be offered an elective Caesarean, as Denise was, and this is especially true if she has had fertility problems. A very high proportion of IVF babies are born by Caesarean section; first, because doctors do not want to put the baby at any risk, and secondly, because the whole pregnancy has become so medicalised that many mothers who could not conceive naturally doubt their ability to give birth naturally too.

This impression is backed up by a study of 195 women having their first baby over 35, compared with another 196 women in the same situation who had a history of infertility. The study showed that the women with no history of infertility had a four-fold risk of pre-term delivery (less than 37 weeks), a five-fold risk of Caesarean section and significantly increased rates of vaginal assisted delivery, chronic hypertension and fibroids when compared with women having their first baby between the ages of 20 and 25. Those who had suffered from infertility had twice as many elective Caesareans as those in the other group, but otherwise there was no difference in outcome.

Unfortunately, in medical litigation cases, inaction can be seen to be negligent while intervention is not, so even if in a particular labour mother and baby's chances would be best served by doing nothing, doctors feel they have to intervene to protect themselves. When a mother is older and her baby is considered a 'precious' baby, intervention is much more likely.

However, mothers who opt for a natural, and particularly, a home birth, do so largely in the belief that it is safer:

'I had my third child at home at the age of 35. I believe – and there is a lot of evidence to support this – that home birth is safer if there are no special risk factors, and the labour was far quicker and in every way better than the previous two. I actually believe that probably more babies die as a result of infections picked up in hospital and mis-managed, extended and messed-around with labour in hospital than would die at home in the rare event that something goes wrong. However, I do accept that at 35 with a first baby I would not have had the confidence to have a home birth, and if I had no children or a history of infertility I would probably feel differently too.'

Marianne, pregnant with her first baby at 39 after two years of infertility treatment, however, disagreed. 'This might be my only baby. I'll do whatever the doctors suggest. I'd like a natural birth, of course, but if things go wrong, if they suggest a Caesarean, I'll go along with it.'

Bridget Baker, an antenatal teacher in East London, says that in her experience older mothers generally feel positive about their labours. 'I think they are more realistic than the younger mothers, they want a baby rather than a wonderful natural childbirth experience.' However, older mothers may have to stand their ground if they are under pressure to allow intervention in the childbirth process and, like all mothers, will have to make a choice. This means finding out what the options are and understanding what labour, both normal and with complications, involves.

The stages of labour

Labour is divided into three clear stages. The first stage is when the muscles of the womb contract increasingly powerfully, pulling open the cervix or neck of the womb to allow the baby's head to come through. The second stage is when you push with the contractions to force the baby out of the womb, and it ends with the birth of the baby. The third stage is the expulsion of the placenta or afterbirth.

Every labour is different for every woman, and that is why it is so difficult for those who have never had a baby to find out what the experience is likely to be like. Labour begins in a number of different ways. Sometimes the first sign is a 'show' – you will see the blood tinged, gelatinous plug that has sealed the entrance to the womb come away. In some women, the waters break first – this can result in a dramatic gush of fluid or it can simply be a slow leak. If the waters leak for more than 24 hours without labour getting well under way it is advisable to contact the doctor or midwife, as once the waters have broken the baby is exposed to infection.

The most common sign that labour is beginning is a cramp-like pain, rather like the onset of the menstrual period, in your lower abdomen or back. You will probably soon feel this pain turn into distinct contractions, which you can feel as a tightening and hardening of the abdomen accompanied by growing discomfort or pain. These contractions differ from the contractions felt throughout the pregnancy only in their greater intensity. As labour progresses, the contractions become stronger and closer together and also last a little longer.

The duration of the early part of labour varies enormously – some women find the contractions continue without becoming too painful for hours or even days. Others find that they build up very rapidly. You are usually asked to report at the hospital when the contractions are about five minutes apart; however, you will know how long it takes you to get to the hospital and you will not want to be travelling if the contractions are very strong and you are in great discomfort, so go when you are ready. Many women prefer to spend the early part of labour at home in familiar surroundings, able to wander around and make a cup of tea and feel that everything is normal. Indeed, the stress of going into hospital too soon has been known to stop a labour which has not got properly under way. If you are having your baby at home, or a 'domino' delivery, (domino stands for domiciliary in out – where your care is with the community midwives who take you into hospital for the delivery, and your hospital stay may be as short as six hours) you will want to phone the midwife as soon as you are sure labour is established.

When you arrive at the hospital the midwife will take some notes, time your contractions, feel your abdomen and listen to the baby's heartbeat and then give you an internal examination to see how far your cervix has dilated. This is usually measured in centimetres; half dilation is 5cm or so and full dilation is approximately 10cm. Some midwives will talk of 'two fingers' dilated – a finger is about equal to a centimetre. Often it takes a lot longer to dilate the first few centimetres than the last, as the contractions at the beginning of labour are not so strong. Some women, especially those who have had babies before, find that they are already well dilated without knowing it when they arrive at the hospital.

Many women find internal examinations during labour very uncomfortable, if not actually painful. Make sure they are done as soon as one contraction is over so that you are not actually being examined during a contraction. Most midwives feel it is important to check how your labour is progressing, but you don't have to have as many as are sometimes suggested and if the labour is obviously progressing fast and well you may not need any at all. If you find an internal too uncomfortable lying on your back, ask the doctor or midwife if she or he can examine you lying on your side. Unless progress is slow, you don't necessarily have to agree to more internal examinations, although this can help check how the labour is going.

When you arrive at the hospital your baby's heartbeat will usually be routinely monitored with an external monitor. This is tied around your tummy with a strap and you will be asked to keep still so your movements do not interfere with the reading. Most women find this very restricting. If all seems well, the monitor will be removed after 20 or 30 minutes – it may be replaced again at some point in the labour just to check that the baby is not distressed.

It is a good idea to tell the staff when you arrive if you have any strong feelings about the way you want the labour conducted. Once it has really got under way, you may find yourself swept along by events. Most hospitals today are aware that women should be given a choice about pain relief and about the position they would like to adopt to deliver the baby. Also raise any queries about episiotomies, clamping and cutting the cord, anything else you wish to know and any other worries you may have. Ideally you will have discussed this with staff beforehand and any strong views should be recorded in your notes.

The first stage

During the first stage of labour, the cervix thins and softens and then dilates to allow the baby's head to pass through the birth canal. When the cervix is fully open it is said to be 10cm dilated, and this marks the transition from the first to the second stage.

Once labour has begun, the contractions tend to become stronger as labour progresses, though they tend not to get closer together than about every three minutes. This means you usually get a break in between to recover from each contraction before the next one begins. Progress is not always uniform; occasionally contractions seem to run into one another, and sometimes a very strong contraction will be followed by a weaker one.

Once the woman is fully dilated, she may experience some strange symptoms; shivering, trembling, sweating, or nausea are all common. Some mothers feel restless and want to change position, often into the position in which they want to deliver the baby. At the end of each contraction the mother may begin to feel that she wants to bear down and begin to push the baby out. When the midwife sees these signals she will probably want to do an internal and check that you are fully dilated. If so, you are ready to begin the second stage. If you are not quite fully dilated, the midwife may ask you to 'pant' during the contractions to help resist the urge to bear down.

The second stage

Most women having an active labour find that the bearing down process is a reflex and that they can't stop themselves. Usually women instinctively know to take a deep breath, lowering the diaphragm and putting pressure on the uterus, though a series of short pushes can be more effective than one long one. An upright or semi-upright position is very helpful in assisting the process; if you are lying down you are actually having to push the baby uphill because of the angle of the birth canal. Most women also instinctively push with each contraction and rest in between.

With each contraction the baby should descend lower into the birth canal. At some point the baby's head will become visible from the outside; this is an exciting moment for a partner or birth companion who is present. The mother can be encouraged to know that the baby is really there and about to be born. Just before the birth the perineum begins to stretch to its widest and this can cause a stretching and stinging sensation. If you seem likely to tear, an episiotomy may be made (see page 146); otherwise the tissues become numb when stretched. Once the baby's head has crowned, it will slip out; another contraction should deliver the shoulders and then the rest of the baby.

When the baby is born it may look strange; puttycoloured, and slimy with vernix and some blood. When the baby draws breath – and usually cries loudly – the colour will change to a healthier pink. If the baby is breathing normally you will be able to hold your baby, discover whether it's a boy or girl, count the fingers and toes and begin to get to know one another. Some mothers will want to put the baby straight to the breast.

The third stage

This is the delivery of the afterbirth. Naturally it may take up to 30 minutes, but usually an injection of syntometrine is given after the baby's head is born to speed up the delivery of the afterbirth, with the aim of reducing the risk of post-partum haemorrhage. Gentle traction may be put on the cord and the midwife may press her hand on your abdomen to assist delivery.

Soon after the birth is a good time to put the baby to the breast for the first time, as research has shown that the sooner after the birth a baby feeds, the more likely breast feeding will be successfully established. In nature, the baby's sucking at the breast helps with delivery of the afterbirth. Not all mothers and babies however are ready for a breast feed so don't feel rushed into things; take time to get to know one another.

Risks for the older mother

Many older women do fear that childbirth will be much riskier for them than for younger women, and riskier for the baby, too. This is true to a certain extent, but recent research has shown that it is not much riskier. Even where much older mothers, in their forties or fifties, are concerned the risks may have been exaggerated. In the past, most older mothers had also had a larger number of children, the birth was more likely to have been unplanned and unwanted, and the mother may have been in poorer health. The fit woman who chooses to have a baby later may well be at lower risk than the figures would lead her to believe.

Modern hospital care and antenatal screening reduce a lot of the risks, and while the safest time to have a baby is still between 20 and 25, a mother in her late thirties who is fit and healthy, eats well and takes care of herself in pregnancy is likely to do as well or better than a younger woman who has not taken care of herself. The number of children you have had and the spacing between them is important too: the risks for the first and fourth or more births are greater than for second or third births, and the risks go up if you have a baby within two years of the previous delivery. If you have had a child before, it doesn't matter how long ago this was; a second birth is still likely to be quicker and easier.

The risk of maternal death in England and Wales is about 0.1 per 1,000. Women of 35 or older have at least five times the risk of death of women aged 20–24, and women of 40 or more at least ten times the risk; however, this still seems a reasonable order of risk for a mother who very much wants a baby.

Part of the greater risks of pregnancy and childbirth for

the older mother is due to the fact that she is more likely to suffer from diabetes, cardiovascular disease and other illnesses which affect pregnancy. If the mother does not suffer from any pre-existing disease, the risks are much lower. However, there are specific risks attached to pregnancy and these tend to increase with age. The risk of hypertension for older mothers increases by about 50 per cent. The risk of pre-eclampsia, haemorrhage following birth and dysfunctional labour (when the cervix does not dilate properly) are more prevalent in women over 35. The incidence of placenta praevia, when the placenta is situated over the entrance to the womb and can therefore come away and cause haemorrhage before or during the birth, or other forms of antepartum haemorrhage, increases with age and with the number of pregnancies – for first time mothers the risk goes up from 3 per cent for those under 25 to 5 per cent for those over 35 and doubles for mothers having a fourth child.

However, it may be true that the higher incidence of dysfunctional labour, Caesarean section and other problems may be caused by obstetric intervention in the older mother. If this baby is a more precious one because of previous infertility problems or because the mother is unlikely to conceive again, then doctors are inclined to intervene on behalf of the baby at a slightly greater risk to the mother. There is an increased risk that if the baby is overdue, the placenta of an older woman will fail sooner than that of a woman in her twenties and fail to nourish the baby properly, so a birth is more likely to be induced. Induction means that labour is more likely to be intensely painful, necessitating pain relief and further intervention. It is also likely to be linked to dysfunctional labour, because the cervix is not yet ready to dilate. The higher rate of

Caesarean section is probably linked more to caution on the part of doctors than to any substantial increase in the real risk to mother or baby.

Statistics show that forceps deliveries and Caesarean sections are more common among older mothers. In 1980 in England and Wales, for those having their first baby, just under 20 per cent of women under 25 had forceps deliveries compared with 29 per cent of women aged 25–34 and 33 per cent of women over 35. The risk of having a Caesarean section for older mothers having their first baby, however, is much greater; only 8 per cent of such mothers under 25 had Caesareans compared with 12 per cent of women aged 25–34 and over 30 per cent of women over 35. Curiously older mothers seemed less likely to end up with episiotomies. While 70 per cent of women under 25 having their first baby had episiotomies and 72 per cent of women aged 25–34, just under 60 per cent of first time mothers over 35 had one. However, this may be simply because more had Caesarean sections!

There is some controversy as to whether older mothers have longer labours than younger women. Some obstetricians have said that they have observed that women over 35 tend to have longer labours, but in 1980 20 per cent of mothers over 35 having first babies had long labours compared with 16 per cent aged 25–34 and 10 per cent aged under 25. This is not an enormous difference.

The other risks faced by older mothers are risks to the baby. Women over 35 have about three times the risk of having a miscarriage and about twice the risk of losing their baby before, during or after the birth. There is also a small increased risk in prematurity for infants of women aged 35–44, but this is only slightly higher than for infants of mothers in their twenties and thirties. One Swedish study

showed that the risk of preterm birth for mothers aged
30–34 was 20 per cent more than in mothers aged 20–24,
from 35–39 was 70 per cent more and over 40 was double.
The rate of low birth weight babies was also about double
for women over 35. There is also, of course, a greater risk
of older mothers having an abnormal baby, and this may be
responsible for some neonatal deaths. A recent US study of
mainly professional first-time mothers over 35 however,
showed no evidence of older mothers being at greater risk
of pre-term delivery, of having a small-for-dates baby or a
baby who died in the peri-natal period.

Pain relief in labour

The pain of labour is very different from other kinds of
pain; it is the pain of your body doing a very hard and labo-
rious job, not the pain of your being in any way harmed or
damaged. However, labour is normally a very painful experience. Many people have tried to gloss around this or give
the impression, that properly prepared and armed with
breathing exercises and the right attitude, you will not feel
pain; this means that many women are taken by surprise
and feel that they have failed when they do experience
intense pain in labour and feel that they need some relief
from it.

It is known that fear and tension can create additional
pain in labour and make it intolerable. If you tense all your
muscles and fight the contractions you will make it much
more difficult for your body to do its job. You need to
think, therefore, of helping your body through the contractions. This thinking is behind the various techniques of
breathing and preparation which are taught to women in

antenatal classes during pregnancy. By accepting the pain and dealing with it many women find that they do not need painkilling drugs which might also interfere with their being in control. For others experiencing a long and difficult labour, painkilling drugs may provide much needed relief.

Breathing techniques

Slow, deep breathing will help you to relax between, and at the beginning and end of contractions. At the height of a contraction, it may help to breath quickly and lightly, taking air into the top part of your lungs only. During the transition between the first and second stages, when you may feel the desire to push the baby out, the midwife may ask you to wait till she is sure the cervix is fully dilated at which time very short, rapid, panting breaths may help you to overcome the desire to push.

Pain-relieving drugs

There are a number of drugs available which can be given to women in labour to relieve pain. They are particularly useful if you are experiencing a very long labour, if the baby is presenting the wrong way (see below) or if you are becoming exhausted. These drugs, however, can pass into the baby's bloodstream and affect the baby, or may affect the progress of the labour. Many women find it useful to wait a little between the moment they first feel that they may want pain relief and deciding to accept it. In the meantime, they may find that the labour is progressing very well that they are nearly ready for the baby to be born. If the progress is slow, however, or there is any problem, they can decide to accept some pain relief.

Gas and air

Nitrous oxide (laughing gas) mixed with oxygen can be very useful at the peak of labour, and it has the advantages that it does not affect the baby, and that you administer it yourself. The gas and air is contained in a large canister and you will be given a mouthpiece or mask through which to inhale it. The idea is that you can breathe it in a minute before the height of a contraction to help you through the most intense part. You may feel very light-headed when you breathe it in, but this will pass as soon as you stop. Some women, however, don't like the woozy sensation it gives them, while others feel ill or are very sick.

Pethidine

This drug, a synthetic equivalent of morphine, acts as a relaxant and reduces anxiety and thus pain; however, not all women find it is an effective form of pain relief. Some find that it makes them feel heavy and out of control without helping the pain much. Pethidine crosses the placenta and can affect the baby, making it drowsy at birth, especially if the drug is given close to delivery (it should be given at least two hours before the baby is born; this means it cannot always be given at the point in the labour when the woman needs it most). Some babies even need resuscitation after the birth and many are sleepy and slow at breast feeding. Pethidine can also make the mother feel sick.

Epidural anaesthesia

An epidural consists of a local anaesthetic which completely numbs the abdomen and legs, thus removing all sensation of contractions. If an epidural is timed just right, it can be allowed to wear off for the second stage so that you can feel and push with each contraction, thus helping the baby out. It seems to have little or no effect on the baby, but the problem is that because some women cannot feel anything they cannot participate in the second stage of labour, which is likely to be prolonged, and the baby is more likely then to be delivered with forceps.

The 1977 National Epidural Survey showed that 70 per cent of mothers who had epidurals for their first birth, and 40 per cent of mothers in second births, ended up with forceps deliveries.

An epidural is injected into the epidural space in the spine between the vertebrae and the membrane enclosing the spinal cord. You will be asked to lie on your left side, pulling your legs up to make as tight a ball as possible to make it easier for the anaesthetist to put the needle into the spine. You will be given a local anaesthetic so you do not feel the tube being inserted; the anaesthetic is then put in. You will feel it like a cold fluid running down your legs. The catheter is left in your back so the epidural can be 'topped up'; you will also normally have a catheter put in to empty your bladder as you will not be able to do this yourself, and a drip set up in case your blood pressure should suddenly fall, as can happen with an epidural.

For some women, an epidural is the answer to a difficult labour:

'I had been in labour for hours, with very strong contractions, but I simply wasn't dilating much. Eventually I was exhausted and felt I couldn't take any more. They offered me an epidural, and I reluctantly accepted. I must say that the effect was wonderful; within a few minutes of them putting it in I was sitting up and chatting to the nurses and felt that I could cope again.'

Epidurals can cause problems, however. In one in five occasions the epidural does not take properly and provides inadequate pain relief, sometimes down one side only. Occasionally – in about one in 100 cases – the needle punctures the membrane enclosing the spinal cord; this means that you are more heavily anaesthetised and can suffer headaches which can last up to a week after the birth. Very rarely, in about one in 100,000 cases, permanent damage can result.

'I hated it. First the anaesthetist had trouble getting it in and in fact a bit of plastic tube broke off and is still floating around somewhere in my spine. Then I had all these tubes and drips set up, and I couldn't get up and walk for hours after the birth. I didn't feel or see the baby born at all because I could feel nothing; I had no idea it would be like that. What's more, because I couldn't push, he was delivered by forceps so now I have all the pain of lots of stitches which I would rather have done without.'

Women having an epidural should be aware that they are often starting off a chain of medical intervention which they might otherwise have done without. On the other hand, if the labour is likely to be a very difficult one, it means that you are spared a lot of pain and are already anaesthetised if the baby has to be delivered by forceps. And if you should need an emergency Caesarean, the epidural will enable you to be awake and avoid a general anaesthetic when your baby is born.

Pudendal block

This is a painkilling injection into the vaginal wall with a special needle if a forceps delivery is necessary, so that you will feel no pain at all. It was common in the days before epidurals but is now rare.

Local anaesthetics are also given if an episiotomy is necessary and for any stitching done afterwards.

TENS
TENS is an experimental form of pain relief which is being offered in some hospitals. TENS stands for transcutaneous nerve stimulation. Electrodes are placed on the woman's body, usually on her back or stomach, and she can regulate the intensity of the current, which can produce a tingling sensation. It is meant to stimulate release of the body's natural painkillers, endorphins. It seems to help some people, but not those that are experiencing a lot of pain in labour.

Difficult labours

Normally the baby is born with the head down facing backwards so that the widest part of the baby's head passes down through the widest part of the pelvis. The baby's head pressing down on the cervix helps it to dilate, and the baby rotates as it is born, helping the body slip out behind the head.

Some babies however, are born in a different position, and this normally causes problems in labour. A posterior presentation means that the baby faces forwards; its spine can press against the mother's as it moves down, causing pain and slowing up labour, and because the widest part of the baby's head is passing through the narrowest part of the pelvis the baby can more easily get stuck here, again prolonging labour and sometimes necessitating use of forceps.

A breech birth occurs when the baby does not turn, so that the head is not born first; breech babies are normally born buttocks first, occasionally feet first. About four births in a hundred are breech. Most breech births are straight-forward, though you are most likely to need intervention, especially in a first birth. Many women are advised to have an epidural; usually the baby's head is delivered with for-ceps to protect it, and you are likely to have an episiotomy to help the baby's head out. If you should need an emer-gency Caesarean, the epidural will already be set up.

Medical intervention

Over the past decade or two, hospitals have increasingly used a variety of techniques which have revolutionised the process of childbirth. Most of these are intended to save lives, and frequently they do. However, many interventions have become routine in some hospitals, thus interfering with the birth process in many mothers who are not at risk. Hospitals are now more likely to discuss any possible intervention with you, and you should make your views clear, although obviously everyone should accept that inter-vention may be necessary in case of an emergency.

Episiotomy

An episiotomy is a small incision made in the perineum, the skin between the vagina and the anus, to enlarge the vagi-nal opening and help the delivery of the baby's head. The cut is made with scissors under a local anaesthetic when the baby's head comes into view. Done properly, the perineum will have stretched very thin and the cut can be made with the minimum of damage and bleeding. An episiotomy should not be necessary in a normal delivery, and you can ask not to have one if you prefer.

However, there is some controversy over whether it is

better to have a small episiotomy or risk tearing the perineum when the baby's head is born. Some feel that a small tear is better and heals more rapidly, others that it is easier to sew up a clean cut. You can certainly ask to be sewn up afterwards by a skilled doctor rather than an unskilled trainee. You should not be in great pain when the stitches are put in; if you are, ask to have more local anaesthetic.

Induction

This is an artificial way of starting labour if it fails to start when all the indications are that the baby is overdue or if there is some need to deliver the baby early. Normally you will not be allowed to go much more than two weeks past your due date if the dates are firm and have been confirmed by ultrasound, as there is some risk that the placenta will not be functioning so well. This is a particular risk in older mothers. Induction doesn't always work; then the mother may be under pressure to have a Caesarean.

'They took me in when the baby was due and said they'd like to induce me. They said that the placenta fails very quickly in older mothers and I was 47. They said there was no sign of placental failure, but that this is a fact. They tried to induce me and it failed. The next day they tried again, but the consultant said, "Let's do a Caesarean, we want a healthy baby." So they did.'

Tests can be done to check that the placenta is working normally and you may also be asked to keep a record of the foetus' movements. If there is evidence that the baby is not growing well, that foetal movements are becoming infrequent or the mother is suffering from high blood pressure, then induction will almost certainly be recommended. Many women are by this time quite willing for the birth to be induced:

'The last few months of pregnancy I was in and out of hospital having tests. I had an agonising pain under the ribs which I knew was caused by the baby but they wanted to check it wasn't something else. I felt incredibly tired – I couldn't cope with the pain and not sleeping – so they decided to induce the birth. I was happy with this. But when I turned up at the clinic they said you're too tired to cope with labour now – go home, rest for a week, don't do anything and if the baby doesn't come we'll induce it next week.'

Labour can be started artificially in several ways. The membranes containing the waters can be broken if the baby is overdue or near to term; this will usually start labour, but if it doesn't other intervention will be needed as there is a risk of infection once the waters have been broken if the baby isn't delivered within 24 hours. An artificial rupture of the membranes (ARM) or amniotomy is performed with an instrument like a long crochet hook. This should be quite painless. The technique is also used to speed up labour as, once the waters have broken, the baby's head, unprotected by the bag of waters, presses harder against the cervix, encouraging the uterus to contract. The contractions will become much stronger and you will also feel some of the waters gushing out with each contraction.

Prostaglandin pessaries are more likely to be used to start off labour. These are usually inserted into the vagina where the effect of the hormones close to the cervix is to trigger labour. A man's sperm contains prostaglandin, which is why women at risk of a premature birth should avoid full sexual intercourse and why one of the best natural ways to induce labour is to make love. A prostaglandin-induced labour works very well because, once started, it can proceed without any further intervention.

If labour does not start in any other way, an oxytocin drip is used. Oxytocin is the hormone which naturally causes the contractions of labour and various artificial forms of it can be used. A drip is inserted into your arm – you can ask that it is put into the arm you use least and that you have a long tube connecting you to the drip so that you can move around and change position as much as possible. The contractions caused when you are on an oxytocin drip are usually stronger, longer and more painful, and you may also find that you are plunged into the height of labour without having time to adjust to gradually increasing contractions, which can make the pain more difficult to cope with. Pain relief is often necessary in these circumstances, and this in itself can lead to further intervention.

Electronic foetal monitoring

Once labour is established, the baby's heartbeat and the strength of your contractions can be measured electronically. It can be very reassuring to be able to hear and actually see throughout the delivery that the baby is well and not in distress, though this can also be checked using an old-fashioned ear trumpet or foetal stethoscope. The disadvantage of electronic foetal monitoring is that you will be attached to a machine during labour and you may feel that it is being paid more attention than you. You will not be free to move around, and sometimes the machines do not work properly. Some women have noticed that the slightest change in the baby's heartbeat will lead to intervention, which may not have been necessary.

There is now evidence, especially from the States, that continuous electronic foetal monitoring does not produce any difference on the outcome of labour as far as the baby's health and safety are concerned, although it results in a higher risk of intervention. However, in any single case where monitoring was not performed and a baby dies the doctor or staff may be sued, so monitoring is almost always done to protect them, even though there may be no evidence to show that it was necessary.

Monitoring can be done with an external monitor strapped to your abdomen. Most women find this very awkward as they have to keep still, and it has a tendency to slip off during a contraction:

'They kept fussing around and trying to put it back on and I couldn't concentrate on what I was doing. Most of the time it wasn't in the right place and you just heard a lot of noise, not the baby's heartbeat.'

An internal monitor works better and is less restricting for the mother. However, the waters must be broken and the cervix at least 2–3 centimetres dilated for this to be attached to the baby's head. A tiny scar like a pinprick will be left after the monitor is removed but it is unlikely to cause the baby much discomfort. In cases where it is thought the baby may be distressed, a blood sample may be taken from the baby's head.

Forceps

Forceps deliveries are carried out when the first stage has been completed and the cervix is fully dilated, but for some reason the baby's head is not coming down the birth canal, or if the baby is in distress and needs to be born rapidly. Premature babies may well be delivered by forceps to spare their heads from being too compressed as they come through the birth canal, and forceps are also usually used to protect the baby's head in a breech birth.

If your baby needs a forceps delivery you will be asked to lie on your back and your legs will be put into stirrups. You will be given a local anaesthetic and an episiotomy will be done to increase the vaginal opening. The forceps will then be gently inserted around the baby's head and gentle pulling will help the head out. Once the head is born the rest of the delivery occurs normally. If the baby's head is facing the wrong way, then forceps may be used to rotate the baby's head to help delivery.

Forceps deliveries are very safe and there is little chance of the baby being harmed in any way, although most will have marks on the head from the forceps for a few days after the birth. Forceps deliveries occur more often after a protracted labour where the mother becomes exhausted, where she has had an epidural and cannot feel to push with each contraction, or where the baby's head is large or in the wrong position.

Sometimes a vacuum extractor, called a ventouse, is used instead of forceps. This is a cup placed on the baby's head operated by a vacuum pump. It can be inserted before the cervix is fully dilated and is used, in conjunction with the mother's pushing, to deliver the baby. A small circular mark where the cup was placed will show on the baby's head for a few days after the delivery.

Caesarean section

Caesarean sections are carried out more frequently than ever before; about one in nine births in the UK is now by Caesarean, and the rate is much higher for older mothers.

The main reason for this change is that the operation has become much safer than previously. Improvements in anaesthetics have lowered the risk, especially since a planned Caesarean can now be done with an epidural rather than general anaesthetic.

The development of the low, transverse 'bikini cut' incision also made the operation safer and more acceptable, and decreased the risk for women who may want to have a later birth the normal way. An influential survey carried out by the organisation Maternity Alliance, One Birth in Nine, which covered 80 per cent of maternity hospitals and one in five obstetricians, gave some disturbing reasons for the increase in the number of Caesareans. The major reasons given were to prevent the stillbirths and deaths of newborn babies by performing Caesareans for breech births, premature and low birth weight babies, and when the baby showed signs of distress. But doctors also said that Caesareans were given because staff were inexperienced in dealing with difficult vaginal deliveries.

The most common reason for a Caesarean is when the baby's head is too big to pass through the pelvis, but other reasons include when the mother is suffering from a disease, such as diabetes or chronic high blood pressure, or when the uterus does not contract properly, even with stimulation, or when the placenta is wrongly positioned (placenta praevia).

The mother's age will also be taken into account, as it is anticipated that older mothers will have more difficult labours and the baby may be more precious, especially if the woman has suffered infertility or miscarriages or may not conceive again. In these circumstances a doctor may prefer to do a Caesarean than take any risk for the baby:

'The staff never mentioned my age at all. I wasn't made

to feel old. It was only at the end when they discovered she was breech that it suddenly came up, because they wanted me to have a Caesarean. They said, "Well, it's your first baby, it's breech, you've had infertility problems and you're 40. This might be your only baby, so you want to be sure that nothing goes wrong."'

What happens during a Caesarean

If you know in advance that you are going to have a Caesarean, you can plan for it. You can choose to have the operation done under an epidural anaesthetic so that you can see and participate in the birth and see or hold your baby as soon as he/she is born. Your husband or partner is also likely to be present for the whole of the operation. You can make plans for the extra support you will need when you come out of hospital. If the operation is done as an emergency, however, you are likely to be given a general anaesthetic as setting up an epidural takes time. Your partner may not be able to be present and you are likely to suffer the after-effects of the anaesthetic, making it more difficult to bond with your new baby.

A Caesarean section usually takes about 45 minutes in all, although the baby is delivered in the first 5–10 minutes, the rest of the operation being the stitching up. The surgeon makes a cut about 12 cm long, usually horizontally and just below the bikini line. He or she then cuts horizontally through the lower part of the uterus, where there are no main blood vessels. The bag of waters may break of its own accord or have to be broken and the fluid is sucked away. The surgeon then puts his/her hands into the uterus and rotates the baby's head so that it appears in the incision. The surgeon helps deliver the baby's head using his/her hands, or sometimes forceps, and an assistant usually pushes on the top part of the uterus. An injection of ergometrine, a drug which makes the uterus contract and stops any bleeding, is given and the rest of the baby is brought out. The placenta is then delivered and the uterus is sewn up, then the abdominal wall.

Although the Caesarean section is a very safe operation, there is always a risk, albeit a slight one, in such surgery. Many women experience quite a lot of postoperative pain and may find that they cannot get comfortable for breast feeding. Mothers often find it takes them longer to bond with their baby because they are feeling so rough in the days following the delivery:

'Having a Caesarean leaves you so incapacitated it takes so much longer to do things for the baby. Everything the baby does makes you feel so uncomfortable – lifting, feeding – and you are tied down with drips and bottles draining the wound for two days. Your mind is geared to you and not to the baby – it is harder to bond. Because of this I so much appreciated the time I had with her at the beginning. The Caesarean was planned, so it was done with an epidural and I was awake. She was born onto me, though I couldn't feel it – I was able to hold her straight away. I was able to think, "This is my baby and no mistake", and the three of us had about one-and-a-half hours together after the birth. Without that I think it would have been really hard.'

The premature delivery

No one knows what causes a premature labour, nor can much be done to prevent it. There are drugs which can be given to try to stop labour, but the success rate is not very high and in any case these drugs may affect the baby.

Multiple pregnancies are more likely to result in the birth of premature and low birth weight babies, especially if the mother is having more than twins.

Prematurity is defined as much in terms of weight as actual age from conception. A distinction is made between babies who are of low birth weight although they are born at the right time – they are known as 'small-for-dates' – and babies who are born too early. About 6 or 7 per cent of babies are born weighing less than 2,500 grams (5½ lb) and these are responsible for a large proportion of infant deaths. All low birth weight babies are likely to have problems in adjusting to life outside the womb and to need special care.

Babies are born 'small-for-dates' for a number of reasons. Sometimes the baby does not grow enough in the last months in the womb because the mother is malnourished, smokes or drinks a lot, suffers from pre-eclampsia or because the placenta is not working properly (placental insufficiency). Twins often do not grow as large as a single baby would, and some babies are small for genetic reasons or because they have some other abnormality. If the baby appears not to be growing well in the last month or so of pregnancy and the woman suffers from pre-eclampsia or placental insufficiency the baby may be induced because it stands a better chance of survival once it has been born.

No one really knows what triggers a premature birth, as the reasons why labour starts normally are very obscure. Occasionally vaginal infections such as gardnerella vaginalis may be involved. Research is being carried out into the reasons for premature delivery and also to find some effective way of delaying labour if this will increase the baby's chances of survival. Drugs can be given to try to prevent premature labour, but these are not always effective and may have unpleasant side-effects.

However, enormous advances have been made in the care of premature and low birth weight babies and today they stand a much better chance of survival. In 1982, 40 per cent of babies weighing 1,000 grams (2 lb) or less survived, 83 per cent of babies weighing between 1,000 and 1,500 grams (2–3 lb) survived, and 95 per cent of babies weighing 1,500–2,000 grams (3–4½ lb) survived. Measured by gestational age, 70 per cent of babies born at 27 or 28 weeks survive, 80 per cent born at 29 weeks survive and over 30 weeks the vast majority will survive – all these figures, of course, applying to babies who are given special care immediately after birth. Tiny babies of as little as 20 weeks have been known to survive, although this is very rare.

It is comforting to know that if your baby is born prematurely, but after the 28-week stage of pregnancy, he or she stands a good chance of survival. However, going into premature labour is an alarming and frightening experience. Most mothers are completely unprepared and fear that their baby will not survive, and this may colour the whole birth process. The experience can be made worse by being in the wrong place:

'George was born at 28-and-a-half weeks. We had been on holiday when my waters started to leak, so went to the nearest cottage hospital where they really didn't have a clue about anything. We decided that we just had to get back to London where we could have the proper care – I was going to have him at one of the teaching hospitals. I was in a terrible state of anxiety wondering if labour really would start and whether the baby could possibly survive. Once we got to London they said that they couldn't stop labour because once the waters have gone the baby is liable to infection. It was my second birth and a normal labour although I was advised not to have any pain relief as this would affect baby and make his chances poorer.

'He spent weeks in special care, coming home just before Christmas. I was terrified the whole time that he wouldn't make it, and in fact one of the other babies in the neonatal unit who was born at the same time as George died while we were there. It was terrible; I just kept thinking, "That could be me, that could be me."'

Premature babies are not ready to live in the environment outside the womb. The layer of fat under the skin has not been laid down, so the premature baby cannot control his body temperature. Many preterm babies suffer from the respiratory distress syndrome. Their lungs do not contain enough of a substance called surfactant which is necessary for getting enough oxygen. The baby has to make an enormous effort to breathe and without help will rapidly become exhausted. Such babies will need to be given oxygen through a tiny tube down the nostrils or through a face mask; or a mechanical ventilator, which does the work of breathing for the baby, can be used if the baby is in real difficulty.

Some low birth weight babies have low blood sugar; this can also happen if the mother is diabetic or if the delivery was a difficult one. An intravenous drip may be set up to give the baby enough nourishment.

Many premature babies suffer from jaundice. About half of all babies develop mild jaundice, in fact, as a newborn baby has a surplus of red blood cells which are broken down after birth, producing a substance called bilirubin. The baby's liver sometimes cannot cope with the bilirubin rapidly enough and the baby becomes jaundiced. If a baby is very jaundiced, photo therapy can be used to help the body cope. The baby's eyes are covered and the body is illuminated with a light which breaks down the pigments in the body so that the baby can excrete them in its urine.

Almost all premature and low birth weight babies will need to be kept in an incubator. This regulates the baby's temperature and enables the medical staff to give any treatment that is necessary. However, it can be very hard for the mother to relate to her baby if he or she is in an incubator, especially if surrounded by special tubes and equipment. Feeding can also be a problem. All premature babies should be given breast milk if at all possible, as it contains antibodies and other factors which will help the baby fight infection, but the baby may be unable to suck. Some babies who are too weak to breast feed may be able to suck from a bottle filled with expressed milk or from a cup. Others may need to be fed through a tube. However, the mother of a premature baby will usually be shown how to express breast milk to provide for and nourish the baby and to establish her milk supply for when the baby is well:

'It was quite a business, going to the hospital all the time and expressing milk – I found it too difficult to express much at home, although I did this too. But the staff were wonderfully supportive and it made me feel as if I was really helping, was really giving him something no one else could. But it's hard, because though he's home now he's been too weak to feed from the breast and is used to the bottle, and I don't feel I can go on expressing for ever, so I don't suppose I will establish proper breast feeding, though I'll give it a try.'

Some mothers cannot cope with this:

'I couldn't express my milk because all the time he was so ill, I thought he was going to die. It made me so unhappy to express milk I thought he'd never take that I couldn't go on with it.'

Very small babies may look tiny, fragile, even ugly little creatures to begin with, which may make relating to them more difficult. The cry of a premature baby may sound more like the bleat of a lamb or mew of a kitten and many babies are so thin they look more like fledgling birds:

'She was so tiny I couldn't believe it – she weighed only two-and-a-half pounds. She hardly looked human at all, like a little bird that had been pushed out of the nest. Because she had breathing difficulties her little chest heaved and she made funny wheezing noises. She was surrounded with tubes and I wasn't allowed to hold her, so I felt completely unable to relate to her at all.'

But despite their initial problems, the great majority of premature babies will thrive and eventually make up the time lost to them. It is important for the parents to remember, though, that their baby is really the age from the time he should have been born not his actual birthday. One mother explains:

'Since he was born three months early, it was terribly difficult explaining to people. At six months from his birthday, he was of course at the stage of a normal three-month-old baby. If I said to people, he's six months old, they would tut-tut and obviously think he was backward. So in the end I gave his age from the due date, not his birthday to casual contacts. And it was very odd celebrating his first birthday when he was just like a nine-month-old.'

By the second or third birthday, of course, the difference between the baby's age and the developmental stage has narrowed and become unimportant – the baby has 'caught up'.

Stillbirth

The death of a baby is a traumatic experience and one which staff in hospitals may find it difficult to deal with.

They are geared up to dealing with the joy of birth and not the tragedy of death. At the time, doctors and nurses may be taken up with dealing with the aftermath of the delivery or in trying to save a baby's life and have little time for the mother and father, leaving both in a state of uncertainty:

'The delivery was ghastly and he was rushed off to special care the moment he was born. I remember they were all fussing around giving me stitches and cleaning me up, but nobody mentioned the baby. I just assumed he was dead; at first I couldn't believe it, I felt numb, then I started crying. Nobody said anything to me and my husband went off to find someone who would tell him what was going on. Then they came to take me back to the ward and I said, in tears, "I'm not going, I'm not going to the ward to see those mothers and babies." "Why not?" they asked. "Because my baby's dead!" I bawled. At that there was a flurry and someone came to say he wasn't dead at all he was in intensive care but they were sure he'd be all right and I could go back and look at him later. It was, in fact, touch and go, but they didn't say so at the time.'

If a woman is kept uninformed and uninvolved, the consequences can be quite tragic:

'It was obvious that something was wrong as soon as he was born and he was taken to the special care unit. There was some confusion over what different doctors said about whether he would live or not and I found that hard, as I didn't know whether there was hope; meanwhile I was in the normal ward with mothers and babies. I wasn't there when they disconnected the life-support system and let him die – there was no point in doing anything. If I had been more involved and helped by them I think I would have chosen to be with him and to have held him when he died.'

There are probably many women who would have very

similar feelings and reactions. Until very recently parents were not encouraged even to see their baby, who was whisked away as soon as it was confirmed that it was dead. Now, however, hospitals are increasingly aware that many parents want to see their baby and accept its death and have some time to grieve. This applies even if the baby is born with some congenital abnormality; the imaginings of someone who has given birth to an abnormal baby are likely to be much worse than the reality, and again, seeing, being with, and holding the child can help parents to accept:

'They said the baby was deformed and I didn't want to see. But my husband did, and he said, really it's all right, she's quite beautiful, you can look. They had wrapped her up so that her face and arms and tiny feet showed and she was very beautiful, and her face had a peaceful expression that made me at once feel much better about her death.'

A mother whose baby has died can ask not to go to the postnatal ward, but be given a room of her own or perhaps go to the general gynaecological ward. Hormones can be given to suppress the milk supply, though this is less usual now as they can have side-effects; the mother may continue to produce milk for some days, to her great distress. The mother whose baby has died will have all the usual hormonal and emotional changes following a birth, but no baby; she is in a kind of limbo, neither a mother nor not a mother.

If the baby has died due to some lack of intervention or action by medical staff, parents usually take out their anger on the hospital and this can make the situation worse immediately after the baby has died: 'They should have picked up that he was in distress, I can't forgive them.' Anger is a normal part of the grieving process, and being able to blame someone can help make the situation seem more bearable for the parents in the short term. Most stillbirth or neonatal deaths, however, could not have been prevented and blaming hospitals will not bring back a baby who has died.

How the hospital staff deal with a tragedy can make an enormous difference to the experience, so if you do have any worries it can help to talk to them in advance about what you would like to happen in the event of the baby's death, even if this sounds as if you are being unnecessarily morbid:

'I told them that if the baby was dead I didn't want them to whisk her away, I would like to see and hold the baby straight away and deal with my emotions then and there. They brushed this aside and said, of course nothing will go wrong – and of course my baby was born perfectly healthy. But I felt it was important for me to say what I wanted in case the unthinkable happened, so we knew where we stood and I wouldn't be faced with half truths or well-meaning attempts to protect me from reality.'

Women – and men – who have experienced the death of a baby are often told by doctors, hospital staff, relatives and friends to 'forget about the experience – you'll soon have another one'. This is very distressing for the parents who need to acknowledge the death and mourn the loss of their baby before going on to another pregnancy. Some hospitals will help the parents by encouraging them to see and hold the baby, perhaps taking a photograph which they can keep, and discussing what sort of funeral arrangements should be made. Hospitals usually arrange for a cremation or burial free of charge, but some parents find they hastily go along with such arrangements and later are distressed because they did not attend a ceremony and the baby is buried with others or in an unmarked grave.

You will also need to register the baby's birth or death – if the baby was born dead there is a special stillbirth register, and you can ask that the baby's name is recorded so that he or she can be acknowledged as your child, a real individual, and not just 'a baby'. If you feel the hospital is not paying attention to your wishes, be firm and ask for what you want; it may help you feel a lot better about the experience when you look back on it and help you in the natural process of grieving.

Bonding with your baby

Much emphasis has been placed on the importance of mothers bonding with their new baby. It is sometimes described as if 'bonding' is some mystical process which must take place in the early moments after the birth or at least within the first few days or the mother and child relationship will be in trouble. The process of bonding with a child is a very important one, but everyone is different. Some people will fall in love with their future husbands at first sight, others build a relationship slowly over the years. In the end the quality of love achieved may not have much to do with the feelings you felt at first; it is the same with a baby.

There is no doubt, though, that the nature of the delivery and the conditions at the time of the birth can help the mother relate to her baby, or hinder her. Hospitals have on the whole changed enormously in this respect:

'My first baby, whom I had in my twenties, was born in the way it was always done; my husband wasn't there; I did what I was told. The midwife delivered the baby and I just happened to be there. The baby was taken away and bathed as soon as she was born and I was given this clean white bundle to look at. We only saw the babies at feeding time, every four hours, and I had to struggle to breast feed. My husband only saw his child hours later at visiting time.

'With this baby it was complete different. Not only was Peter there the birth, he'd come along for tests and things throughout the pregnancy. It was a pleasant room with pretty wallpaper and curtains, and we could take our own things with us. The birth was fine, although I had a massive haemorrhage afterwards and the baby needed resuscitation – but as soon as all that had been seen to they left us, melted away and turned down the lights and we were left on our own with the soft lighting, pretty wallpaper and music!'

Nowadays most mothers who breast feed their baby will be allowed or encouraged to put the baby to the breast soon after the birth. The baby may be delivered straight onto the mother's tummy and in any case, both parents are likely to be able to see and hold him immediately before he is washed and weighed. Despite this kind of care, however, not all mothers feel a rush of love:

'It was a perfect birth, I saw him born, they delivered him onto my tummy, and there he was, a perfect, beautiful baby with wide open eyes; he didn't yell but looked all round him. I didn't feel a thing – in fact, at this greatest moment of my life, all I said was, "Is that my baby?" I was completely exhausted and drained of any emotion. My husband held him while I was stitched up – I'm sure he bonded with him, because I could hear this long conversation going on, my husband talking to him and gazing up at his face. Then they put him to the breast, but again I didn't feel anything. It was a strange blur.

'Afterwards, when I was on the wards, I would look at

this tiny baby next to me and think, this is it, you should be overjoyed, this is your perfect baby. And to tell the truth, I don't think I did really love him. I mothered him, and did everything I should, felt protective and concerned, but only now he's a person and walking and starting to talk can I say that I really love him.'

Nonetheless, the importance of the early time after the birth must not be underestimated. It can be important to have a time of peace and quietness together before being plunged into all the problems and worries of parenting. The time immediately after the birth provides a perfect time for this. To begin with, the baby is usually awake and alert and not yet frantic to feed. The parents can hold and talk to him and feel that he is really theirs. There need be no other distractions at this time and tasks like bathing the baby, and tidying up the mother can wait. It is a unique moment which should be exploited to the full. Some studies have shown that mothers who have been separated from their babies immediately after the birth find it more difficult to bond, and this does seem to be true of women who have had Caesarean sections or whose babies have had special care. But there are other factors as well. Women who have had infertility problems or have suffered the loss of a baby may have blocked off their emotions in case they do not get their longed-for baby; it can be more difficult to let these emotions out when the baby becomes a reality:

'I had taken a long time to conceive and also had a miscarriage. I began to think that I would never have a baby. When he was born, I think I felt that I couldn't just switch on the love which I'd been bottling up all those years. I had to take time to get used to the fact that this was real and to get to know him.'

Some women find that being in hospital makes it more difficult for them to relate to their babies. With all the activity going on, the streams of visitors to yourself and other mothers, the comings and goings of doctors and nurses, there can seem to be little time alone to get to know your baby. Worse, your partner can only visit and when he is with you there is little privacy:

'On the fourth day I had the blues that everyone seems to have, when your milk comes in and your hormones are all upside down. I felt I couldn't cope so I went and hid in a room off the nursery to have a good cry. Then some mother came to find me and said, "Your baby's screaming its head off, what are you doing?" So I went back to feed the baby. She came with me and I know she was trying to help, she said, "Oh, we've all had the weeps, don't worry about it." But she kept making comments about how I was feeding the baby. I just wanted to be alone, and I wanted my husband there, especially at nights. I would lie awake at nights wanting just to cuddle him and when he did come of course all I could get was a peck on the cheek with everyone else around.'

Many women feel that the time after the birth should be one for them and their families alone:

'Despite having a Caesarean I left after six days in hospital. They said you shouldn't be leaving but I wanted the three of us to be together – I thought we'd muddle through better than here where there's all this help, that is clinical and not emotional.'

'I came home after one day because I didn't want my little boy to come and see us in hospital. I didn't want him to find me stuck in a strange hospital bed and the baby in a plastic crib and unable to be ourselves. I thought he should see us all at home and get to know the baby there, to have his mother with him and not to have to go away and leave us in a strange place.'

Today it is normally accepted that the father will be present at the birth of the child. This is one of the greatest changes that has taken place in the last few decades of child-bearing practice, although, before hospital births became the norm, many fathers would have been present at home for their child's birth. Few hospitals make any objection to the father's presence even at difficult births like forceps deliveries or Caesareans, and the father is often involved in holding the baby after the birth while the mother is stitched or cleaned up and while the afterbirth is delivered. Visiting hours have also been made more flexible so that at most hospitals fathers have unlimited visiting and can get to know their child a little before they are all at home together.

A great many fathers find the whole experience of birth exciting and rewarding and say they feel closer to their children because of it. Others may also feel that they were helpless and couldn't do anything to prevent their partner's suffering which they found very upsetting. Not all men provide the help expected:

'He went green and looked terrible. I really felt for him, it made it worse for me in a way. I kept thinking I just can't yell, it'll upset him too much.

'At the worst stage in the labour I asked him how he was feeling and he said, "I'd rather be at home in bed." I think he just felt helpless. I felt really betrayed by him, that he could be so insensitive at that moment – but then he finds it very hard to show his feelings and he had to put on a masculine front.'

'They offered me pain relief and I decided to take it, despite our plans for a natural birth. But he refused to let me take anything. He kept telling the staff, "She doesn't mean it, she's OK." In a way I'm pleased in retrospect, but at the time I thought, "What does he know about how I am feeling?"'

Other women feel that they could not have managed without their partners:

'He was wonderful. It helped knowing he was there and he really soothed me. When the baby was born he was so thrilled, he was beside himself. He was holding the baby as soon as they would give him to him – I wouldn't have had him miss out on that for the world.'

Where the father is unable or unwilling to attend, most hospitals will allow you to have a close friend or relative as your birth partner to provide support and help. Sometimes the hospital staff seem to discourage an early discharge because they feel you will be unsupported at home. This is often not the case; many women find that they can relax and solve problems once they have sole charge of the baby and do not feel they have to get permission all the time to do what they feel most comfortable.

However, there has been a steady trend towards women going home from hospitals earlier. The once accepted, two-week stay has gone down to an average of four or five days, and the majority of women with no problems are now discharged after 24–48 hours.

Breast feeding

The majority of women leaving hospital today are breast feeding their babies. This is especially true for middle-class and professional women, among whom the majority of older mothers are likely to be. Age does not seem to have any great effect on breast feeding; it is not commonly known that any woman who has had a baby can breast feed, and that in other cultures grandmothers breast feed their daughter's children. Occasionally a much older mother may find it a problem to produce enough milk, due to hormonal problems, but this is very rare.

Many hospitals now give great support and encouragement to mothers who want to breast feed, recognising that it is the best food for a baby and that there are emotional rewards for the nursing mother. But some women decide that they do not want to breast feed and there is no reason why they should feel guilty about this as there are excellent artificial baby milks now available which are made to match the mother's milk as closely as possible from the nutritional point of view. Bottle-fed babies also thrive and love is more important than the way you choose to feed, though many mothers choose to express their love through breast feeding.

Breast feeding is best for a baby because it is a living substance transmitted direct from mother to baby, containing white blood cells, antibodies and other substances which help protect the baby against disease. It is composed of exactly the right nutrients for human babies and is produced in the right quantities demanded by the baby. After the birth a mother produces colostrum – a yellowish fluid rich in antibodies which protects the baby from infection. It also contains protein, water and minerals in just the right proportion for the baby's first few days, and a natural laxative which helps the baby's bowels to get moving. When the milk comes in it is also perfectly balanced for the baby's needs. The milk changes slightly in composition as the baby grows, and research has shown that milk produced by the mothers of premature babies is different from the normal milk, and ideally suited for them.

When the baby first goes to the breast and sucks it takes the watery foremilk stored in ducts behind the areola, the pigmented area around the nipple. The baby's sucking sends a message to the brain to let down the bulk of the milk, and the hormone oxytocin – the same hormone which makes the womb contract in labour and at orgasm – is released, causing the muscles around the glands producing the milk to contact and squeeze the milk through the breast to the nipple. The baby usually takes the bulk of the feed in the first ten minutes or so at the breast, but milk is always produced so the feed can last much longer than this.

Most hospitals have made-up bottles of formula readily available and this is a great temptation to a mother who is having problems with breast feeding and who is very tired. If you are keen to breast feed do resist this temptation. It takes some time to establish breast feeding and there are often initial problems, but they should sort themselves out. Some babies used to the bottle find it more difficult to take the breast, and babies who have had bottles sometimes reject the breast altogether. Mothers who are keen to avoid cow's milk because of eczema and asthma in the family should also resist the temptation to give a bottle.

Starting feeding

It is important to feel comfortable and relaxed when you are breast feeding. Get into a position which puts no strain on your back, shoulders or limbs and hold the baby comfortably, perhaps resting on a pillow so he is at the right height. Use his 'rooting' reflex to get him to feed – brush the cheek nearest the breast and he will turn his head, mouth open, to latch on.

It is very important to see that the baby has a large part of the areola, the area around the nipple, in the lower part of his mouth. If he has just the nipple you will soon become terribly sore and he will not be able to get the milk out. Once he is latched on and feeding properly, you should not feel great discomfort, even if your nipples are sore. If you do feel any pain, remove his mouth by slipping your little finger in the corner of his mouth to break the suction, and try again.

At the end of the feed the baby is likely to be sucking very gently for comfort only and if this is sending him to sleep there seems to be little point in removing him till he is satisfied. If your nipples are sore or if you are tired or need to do something else, don't feel guilty about removing him.

Because breast feeding does not come naturally to the majority of women and because it is easy to be put off by initial difficulties, many mothers need a great deal of support to establish breast feeding, particularly after a Caesarean:

'The most difficult time was the first few weeks. Because I couldn't exclusively feed him I had to supplement, which was very disappointing. I did everything under the sun to try and get him to breast feed exclusively. I had a lot of support but because of the Caesarean I had an infection and had to take antibiotics which were not compatible with breast feeding and which I didn't question at the time, although I should have done. This all militated against breast feeding and, of course, they put him on formula straight away in hospital which again I would question if I had to go through it again. We got through it, but it was a very difficult time. I think because I was older that I should have known how to cope – that somehow I shouldn't have felt so demoralised in those first few weeks.'

With other difficulties to overcome the initial experience may be unrewarding as well as discouraging. And it may take time and a lot of encouragement to get over these hurdles:

'After a Caesarean I suppose I had a bad start in establishing breast feeding and now she's six-weeks-old or so we have only just sorted them out. They said after a Caesar it takes longer for the milk to come in and it's difficult to hold a baby when you're feeling so sore. Also my breasts were so painful – the nipples so sore – nobody had prepared me for that. I kept thinking, "Where is this wonderful experience? Am I normal?" Finally, it was talking to a relative which helped – she said, "Yes, it is painful but it will get better." I think in a way I had too much information and advice – I changed to the bottle as the midwife advised it and then went back to the breast – I just needed someone to say, "yes, it is awful at the beginning and I've been through it and it does get rewarding in the end".'

Many women are given the impression that they must either totally breast feed or bottle-feed and there is no 'in between'. While it may be true that it is important to breast feed entirely for the early weeks while you are building up a good supply, the odd 'relief bottle' which a partner or childminder can give can be a great bonus and prevent a mother from giving up entirely:

'I only breast fed for six weeks. I found it too demanding – she never lasted for two hours and wanted feeding all the time. No one said you could breast and bottle-feed. So I just stopped and put her on a bottle which she took quite well. I didn't ask advice from the health visitor – I didn't get on with her. I'd feel all right until I saw her and then she'd upset me – that didn't help. At the baby clinic I had to wait so long I didn't bother.'

Even if you are going back to work quite soon after the birth, breast feeding for the first few weeks gives the baby the best possible start and you can continue to breast feed morning and night if you choose.

Breast feeding is a completely different experience to bottle-feeding and cannot be fitted into the idea of strict schedules and routines which were prevalent a generation ago. Breast feeding mothers, who know they should feed on demand and as often as every two hours if the baby wants it, find it annoying and discouraging to hear others say, 'You can't be feeding him again, surely?' The frequent lack of understanding among older relatives and friends and even professionals means that many mothers are discouraged needlessly from breast feeding in the early weeks. Support groups like the National Childbirth Trust (NCT) and the Laleche League can be very helpful. Most local NCT groups have a breast feeding counsellor who can help mothers with any worries or problems.

If you do have problems, try to persevere. Apart from the physical advantages of breast feeding for the baby, it offers a unique bond of closeness between mother and baby once initial problems have been overcome:

'I simply can't imagine not having fed my baby myself. It was the most wonderful thing that whenever I was exhausted or she was fretful we could just sit down and relax and be totally absorbed in one another. It was so easy, so natural, and made me at once feel at peace with myself and the baby . . . even at four a.m., it was easy just to pick her up and latch her on and sometimes I would doze back to sleep, too. And it was a wonderful feeling as she grew to feel that I had done it all myself.'

Breast feeding: problems and solutions

Sore nipples

In the early days the nipples may become sore and painful. You may get small blisters and sores. Very sore, puffy red nipples may be caused by thrush which can also affect the baby.

It is important to check that the baby has its mouth open wide enough and is not tugging on the nipple. Sunlight and fresh air help sore nipples heal and you can rub a little expressed breast milk on them. Cream can be prescribed for thrush.

Cracked nipples

If the baby is poorly latched on a crack can occur in the nipple – this is very painful and it may bleed.

If you latch the baby on properly you can still feed from a cracked nipple. You may need to express milk from that breast for 24 hours to allow the crack to heal.

Engorged breasts

This often happens when the milk first comes in before the baby gets feeding established. If the breasts are too full the areola can become too hard for the baby to latch on properly and a vicious circle then results.

Expressing some milk before a feed softens the breast and helps the baby to latch on properly. Hot flannels or a bath will relieve the breasts, or you can use cabbage leaves inside your nursing bra.

Blocked duct

You may notice a hard lump in one breast and that the breast seems engorged above it. If the blockage doesn't clear, the patch may become red and infected – mastitis can result, in which the breast becomes red and you run a high temperature. It is important to go on feeding the baby; if you stop the mastitis will get worse.

Put the baby to the blocked breast first and try to position him so that his lower jaw is where the blocked duct is. Massage the breast towards the nipple and use hot flannels before a feed. If mastitis results, carry on feeding, and see a doctor for antibiotics.

Breast abscess

If mastitis does not clear you may get a breast abscess. If you carry on feeding through mastitis this is very rare.

You will need to see a doctor to have the abscess dealt with through aspiration or surgery. You can usually continue to feed the baby, and certainly can from the unaffected breast.

The postnatal check

Six weeks after the birth you will return to the hospital or your GP for a check-up to ensure that your body is returning to normal after the birth. The doctor will feel your abdomen to check that the womb has returned to its normal size. Your blood pressure and weight will also be noted. You will be asked if you have had any unusual bleeding, pain or discomfort. (It is quite common for the lochia – the blood loss after the birth – to continue for more than six weeks, and some women have already had a period by this time.) Any scars from tears or episiotomies will be checked and your breasts and nipples may be examined if you have problems with breast feeding.

You may also discuss contraception with your doctor if this has not already been arranged. Women who use a diaphragm will usually have it refitted at the postnatal check, although everything may not have returned to its normal shape and size and it may need checking again a few weeks later. An IUD can also be refitted at six weeks – it cannot usually be done immediately after the birth because there the womb is still contracting in size and may expel the device. If you want to take the pill, the usual combined oestrogen/progestogen pill is not suitable if you are breast feeding as it affects the milk supply. The mini-pill or progestogen-only pill can be taken within seven days of the birth, although some mothers do not like the idea of taking any drug while breast feeding, and it is known that small quantities of hormones do get through to the baby though there is no evidence to date that this is harmful. Many couples rely on the sheath as a temporary measure as it really is an ideal method at this time.

You will have the opportunity to raise any worries you have about your own health or that of the baby, including problems with breast feeding. You may like to discuss problems you have with sex, especially if you have attempted intercourse and found it painful. It is very common not to have had sexual intercourse till after this postnatal stage – indeed, many women find that they need the reassurance of the postnatal check that all is well before they do so.

If you did not have a cervical smear taken earlier in pregnancy, now is a good time to have it done.

6

Adjusting to parenthood

The early days

The transition to parenthood is one of the greatest changes anyone will experience, yet most parents are unprepared for it. Often the pregnant woman and her partner focus on the birth itself as the end of pregnancy rather than caring for the baby. While antenatal classes may foster this problem, many antenatal teachers say they find that some pregnant women simply cannot see beyond the birth. They know they're going to have a baby, but they just can't visualise it or imagine what it's like.

You've finally had the long-expected baby. Labour is over, whether it went well or badly, and you are holding the child in your arms. What do you feel? Overwhelming love for this new person? Elation, joy, relief? Shock and disbelief – is this baby really mine? How will I cope? Doubt and fear – Can I cope? Do I want this baby?

Most new mothers probably feel a mixture of all these feelings, but we are only supposed to acknowledge the first. To begin with, many women feel a sense of elation that they have given birth, especially if the labour has gone well.

They may feel a real 'high', showing the baby off to everyone, making lots of telephone calls to tell everyone the
good news. After this 'high' may well come a feeling of
exhaustion, of sudden flatness, weepiness and confusion;
the classic 'four-day blues'. This may also be caused by
hormonal changes as the level of pregnancy hormones
drops away and as the mother's milk comes in.

Mothers may experience very strong physical reactions
after labour. 'It was a long labour, and I was completely
exhausted', recalls Wendy, who had her first baby at 35. 'I
remember lying in the hospital bed and being afraid that I
couldn't breathe.' Gill found that she trembled uncontrol-
lably for hours after the delivery. New mothers often have
stitches, are stiff from the exertions of labour and perhaps
squatting or crouching for long periods, have tender tum-
mies and sore breasts, and lack sleep.

Pauline says, 'I expected everything to be different, but I
couldn't have imagined how different. After three days in
hospital my partner drove me home with the new baby. I
was driving through London and everything looked more
clear and sharp than ever before, as if I was seeing it differently, almost as if I was on drugs or something.'

Some mothers experience a profound feeling of unease,
directed at the baby: Will he be all right? Will he go on
breathing? Together with this is fear about whether the
baby will thrive. Breast feeding often causes a great deal of
anxiety: Is the baby still hungry? Is there enough milk? Are
the breasts or nipples the right shape? How often should
one feed?

Many mothers remember the first few days at home with
a new baby as a strange, timeless period, in which the
mother spends a lot of time in bed and in the tasks of holding, changing, and feeding the baby. Often the new mother

has some help for the first week or so; the partner has time off work, a mother or mother-in-law comes to help.

If the labour has been long, difficult, and not ended as the mother hoped, perhaps with a Caesarean section, the mother may initially feel depressed and have strong feelings of failure, which may colour her initial reaction to the baby and to motherhood. A badly conducted labour, in which the mother feels control has been taken away from her and in which frightening and unpleasant procedures are carried out, can be a shocking experience, especially because the mother may be fearing something will go wrong for her baby.

No sooner has labour ended than the new mother is plunged into the relentless task of caring for her baby, day and night. Sally, a first time mother at 36, says 'What's hardest is getting used to being useless at something again. At this age, you're used to being good at what you do – at your job, socially, running a home – when suddenly this baby comes along and you haven't a clue how to look after it. If I were 24, I would take learning something so new more in my stride.'

Another older mother recalls her feelings of horror when she realised what lay in store for her: 'I remember thinking 24 hours after he was born, "*What have I done?*"' One older mother remembers putting her baby down in the carry-cot in the centre of the room and then sitting down and crying. 'What was I to do with him? I would have to wake up two or three times a night every night from now on. I could never go anywhere without him, or if I did, I would have to rush back again soon and I would worry about him all the time anyway. *Nothing was ever going to be the same again.*'

Other mothers, despite the usual anxieties and stresses of

adjusting to the new baby, recall the few weeks after the baby's birth as a very special, intense, thrilling time in their lives. 'I felt so pleased with myself,' says Fiona, 38. 'I had produced this perfect baby, and she seemed to thrive in my care. I loved the fact that she depended on me totally, I felt really important to someone for the first time in my life. There wasn't anything I'd rather do.'

Settling down

After the initial 'honeymoon' period, where the mother usually has help and the admiration of friends and family, life goes back to 'normal' – except that it is nothing like the life the mother used to lead. For some this is positive, others – and perhaps the majority – feel far more ambivalence. Many first time older mothers describe the birth of their first child as 'opening a whole new chapter' in their lives:

'You can't be alone. I miss my freedom, I miss the privacy,' says one mother who is on her own with the baby, often all day long. Her whole time is taken up with the routine tasks of feeding, changing and pacifying the baby. When the baby sleeps, she uses the opportunity either to tidy up the home or to snatch a short period of much needed sleep to make up for the deprivations of the night.

'I feel like a zombie. Midday comes, and I still haven't got dressed. I feel too tired to do anything. I can't cope with the housework, I just don't care about it and I don't want to do it, but if the place got to be a mess I just feel too depressed.'

Zoë had twins at the age of 38. 'My husband came home once and told me off because I hadn't watered the houseplants, which were wilting. I had to go to a meeting and he took the afternoon off to look after the twins. When I came back I asked him if he'd had time to water the plants and he had to admit that he hadn't. I think that one afternoon showed him a little bit of what I was going through.'

Older mothers who have waited a long time to have a baby, especially those who have had fertility problems, may be horrified to find that once they have had the baby they do not feel overjoyed. 'I did at first – for a few days. Then this sort of depression set in. I was so tired, I couldn't cope, I didn't feel anything very much towards this baby, he was just a red-faced little creature who cried a lot. I couldn't bear to admit to myself that this wasn't wonderful. How could I have gone through three years of infertility treatment, IVF and a miscarriage so that I could be a mother, and then find that I didn't like it?'

This mother only found her equilibrium once she returned to work part-time, six months later.

'I think the thing about becoming a mother is that you instantly become a non-person. You are just a stay-at-home mum with a baby and you don't feel you count for anything.' Claire, 39, who was a microbiologist, stands in her untidy kitchen with an 18-month-old clinging to her leg. She wears an old sweatshirt which is covered in marks left by grubby fingers, no make-up, and hasn't combed her hair. She says 'I feel about as sexy and as intelligent as a potato. My husband changed jobs and I gave up mine, as we were moving, and had a baby, and I spend all day at home with this horrible toddler whining at me and widdling everywhere. I was a highly qualified and respected person at work, and now look at me. When the Chinese communists made intellectuals work on the land and do all kinds of menial tasks Amnesty International said it was an abuse of human rights. Well, why isn't it an abuse of human rights when a highly qualified microbiologist has to wipe widdle off the kitchen floor and read Postman Pat all day long?'

Exhaustion is one of the main complaints of older parents, who simply do not have the resilience of the young person. Linda Kelsey, former editor of *She* magazine, said at 40: 'I do not think women in their fifties realise the physical toll. I felt absolutely exhausted.' Actress Patricia Hodge, who had sons at the age of 42 and 45, said: 'I can't pretend there haven't been times when I've wept from one end of the weekend to the next with sheer exhaustion.'

Some recent research has shown that older men and women are less able to cope with sleep shortages and disruption than younger people. After the age of 40 in particular the amount of time spent in deep sleep decreases. There are more awakenings in the night and sleep itself becomes lighter. As people get older they tend to lose the ability to fall asleep quickly, to sleep during the day or to sleep late to make up for a late or broken night.

As people age, it may be that sleep rhythms get more fixed and it becomes more difficult to adjust the pattern. After years of regularly waking and getting up at seven, it may be harder for people to 'sleep in'. A new baby's pattern of sleeping for short periods may create havoc for the older mother's sleep patterns.

Some older mothers, anxious to avoid the double burden of loneliness and exhaustion, seek paid help in the early weeks. Some hire a nanny or maternity nurse to help with the baby. This can be a great success, and can give the mother help and companionship at a difficult time, but not always. Louise found that the maternity nurse undermined her own confidence and wanted to do things her way:

'It was my first baby and about the fiftieth she'd looked

after. I felt helpless in comparison. Also, she didn't understand that I wanted to breast feed the baby on demand and kept saying he was feeding too frequently. She kept asking if she could give him a bottle so that I could rest; she was obviously frustrated that she couldn't feed him. She fussed around and I didn't feel I could relax. The only helpful thing was when she took the baby for a walk. In the end I told her to go and hired a cleaning lady instead; that was much more useful.'

The crisis of motherhood

Sometimes late motherhood produces a real sense of crisis. Women's fantasies and expectations are not always met by motherhood and they can be confused when they are not able to manage the transition better. 'Before he was born I had the illusion that I would continue my life much as before – going out with friends, to the theatre or concerts, just getting a babysitter when needed. I had no idea that I would be so tired or that the baby would make such demands that this became impossible. I thought the baby wouldn't tie me down and now look at me.'

In an essay called 'Psychotherapy with pregnant women', therapist Joan Raphael-Leff observes that women who come to motherhood later may have consciously set aside, avoided, denied pregnancy during past years. The conflicting emotions from these earlier years will still be in the subconscious. When they have the baby, these may then resurface, causing conflict.

Older mothers are more likely than younger ones to have reached a point where their lives are ordered and they have things running much as they wish. The arrival of a new baby can upset all these routines and precipitate a chaos the mother cannot cope with. The transition from being an autonomous person to someone who is constantly at the receiving end of demands from the infant can be overwhelming. And the problem is, it's inescapable. 'People kept saying to me, why don't you go out and leave the baby for an afternoon or evening. But that was just the point. I didn't want to leave her; I couldn't bear to be separated from her for an instant. It was the tyranny of my own emotions I couldn't escape from, not her.'

The birth of a second baby can present almost more problems than the first. Statistics show that the trend to late motherhood has also shortened the space between births; if the older mother wants to have more than one child she has to squeeze them in quickly. The General Household Surveys of 1988 and 1989 show that women who began childbearing in their 30s had an average of 27 months between their first and second baby and 30 months between second and third as compared with 30 and 35 for mothers in their twenties. The older the mother, the shorter the gap is likely to be.

The arrival of the second baby means that the mother is now much more tied than she was before. While it was possible for her alone or with her partner to pop out for the evening with the baby in a carry-cot, it is almost impossible to do anything spontaneously with a small baby and demanding toddler. 'My day was totally circumscribed,' says Annie, whose children were born when she was 40 and 42. 'I had to stick to my daily routine or it was hell. There were just under 18 months between them. James needed a sleep for an hour after lunch or he was unbearable. He needed feeding at regular times. Everywhere I went I had to take the baby in a sling and the toddler in a pushchair, jars of ready prepared foods, drinks and the like. For nearly a year I had two sets of nappies. By the time the baby was three months old I was so exhausted I didn't know what I was doing and I was so bored I thought I would go mad. If one of them was ill or it poured with rain I just didn't know how I would get through the day.'

There is only one way to survive; the companionship of other mothers. Just someone to talk to, to say how you are feeling, can make all the difference. Unfortunately, older mothers may find it more difficult to meet other mothers in their situation. 'I think there are more older mothers now, but when I had my son ten years ago there weren't so many around,' says Vivienne, who was 41 when her daughter Ruth was born. 'Most of the other mothers I met at antenatal classes were ten years younger and they thought they were 'old' to have a baby at 32! At first we would meet for coffee, but we didn't really have so much in common. I did want to meet other mothers like myself.'

Other mothers found a different experience:

'I didn't think it was very unusual to have babies late. Most of the mothers in my antenatal class were in their thirties and some in their late thirties. There were quite a few late mothers at the local playgroups and I found there was a lot of support. We were all very willing to help one another out.'

Effect on the couple's relationship

The longer a couple have been together before having a baby, the harder it may be to adjust to having a new baby. Research shows that the most stressful and difficult time in a marriage is after the birth of the first baby. 'There's no

doubt that the birth of a baby can rock a marriage,' says
Zelda West-Meads of Relate. The couple suddenly have
much less time for one another and sex often suffers.

Having a baby can completely change the nature of a
couple's relationship. 'Before we had the baby we used to
go out a lot, see friends, we were always doing something.
Suddenly we were both at home, and our worlds completely diverged. He was still out there, doing things,
meeting people, and when he came home all I had to report
on was whether the baby had been particularly fretful or
some possible problem with his health.'

Sex, too, suffers in the weeks and often months after the
birth. Studies have shown that the majority of mothers do
not have sexual intercourse with their partners till at least
six weeks after the birth of the baby; one study showed that
of 119 women, only 35 per cent had made love before the
six week check. This study also showed that over half the
women said they were less interested in sex three months
after the birth than before pregnancy, and by a year after
the birth 57 per cent of women were still not having sex as
often as before.

The delay in resuming sex after the birth is partly for
medical reasons; stitches have to heal, bruising clear up,
there is a possible risk of infection, and the mother often
still has the lochia, the post-childbirth bleeding.
Contraception, too, is an issue; a cap or IUD (coil) cannot
be fitted till six weeks after the birth, and the pill is not
advised because it may reduce the milk supply and hormones are passed through in the breast milk to the baby.
(The mini pill does not affect the milk supply and there is
no evidence that the hormones harm the baby, but the pill
has not been in use long enough for a generation to grow
up and have children themselves, so most mothers are wary

of taking the pill while breast feeding.) Many women –
and their partners – see the six week check as an 'all clear'
to resume sexual relations if all is well.

Most mothers, however, find that their libido is altered
by becoming a mother and that they do not want to have
sex as often as before or even at all. This may be partly
physiological, as a result of the hormone changes following
pregnancy and during breast feeding, it may be partly psychological, and it may also be partly due to exhaustion.

Breast feeding in particular seems to have an effect on
libido. While nursing her baby, the mother has a high level
of a hormone, prolactin, in her body, which helps to suppress ovulation, and this seems to dampen libido and may
also lead to a decrease in vaginal lubrication. This may be
nature's way of making sure that the mother doesn't get
pregnant again too soon and that the baby isn't therefore
displaced from the breast. In hunter-gathering societies, the
oldest kind of social group, it is usual for the baby to be
weaned from the breast when the mother conceives again
and this isn't usually until the first child is three or four
years old, partly because frequent breast feeding acts as a
contraceptive, but also because sexual intercourse is taboo
when the mother is nursing a young baby. In such cultures
breast milk is an important source of protein for the young
child; in some regions of Africa the word for some kinds of
malnutrition means 'baby displaced too soon from the
breast'.

Some mothers say that they find sex and breast feeding
don't mix: 'I would have this tiny delicate baby at my
breast, stroking me with his little hand, and then I'd put
him down and this great hairy male hand would grab me.'
Some women find they do not like having their breasts
touched by their partner while breast feeding: 'I felt that my

breasts were for my baby. If my husband touched them they'd start leaking milk and, because I wasn't the world's greatest milk producer, I'd worry about the milk which was going to waste. I also used to leak milk when I had an orgasm, so we'd always have to have sex just after I'd fed the baby.'

Other mothers find they enjoy the physicality of breast feeding and enjoy sharing it with their partner: 'I had plenty of milk – too much, in fact – so sometimes I'd let Nick have a taste. It was also quite useful sometimes – I'd get him to suck a little to get the milk to let down when I wanted to express some, or if I got overfull and engorged.'

Psychological reasons why the mother may not want sex have to do with her image of her body and of motherhood. This may especially be the case if a mother has had a bad labour. 'I felt as if I had been raped. I had been taken over, manhandled by doctors, and awful things had been done to the most intimate parts of my body. Apart from all the stitches, inside and out, which got infected and took weeks to heal, I felt terribly traumatised. I simply couldn't bear to be touched for months afterwards.'

Others feel that they have lost some of their sexual attractiveness. This may be more true of older mothers, who may find that the stresses of pregnancy and birth take more toll on their body and that it takes longer to get fit again. 'I had put on weight and my tummy was just a flabby empty bag. My breasts had changed shape and I just didn't feel that I could be attractive to my husband.'

Again, other mothers, especially those who have enjoyed a good birth experience, find the opposite. 'I felt I was really a woman now – my breasts were large and full of milk, I went back to my original weight very soon after the birth, and I felt really sexy and fulfilled. Perhaps that was also because my partner made it clear that he found me very exciting and sexy as a mother.'

Many partners do not understand if the woman has lost interest in sex. Many, especially if they have not had sex at all in the late months of pregnancy and in the weeks after the baby is born, do not see why after a couple of months their sex life should not get back to normal. This can clearly be a cause of strain in the relationship. The important thing is to talk about it and get it out in the open, rather than bottling up the feelings.

Some mothers find that, though they initially may not feel like sex, this is very important for their partner and make the effort:

'I never felt like making love, with a new baby and a demanding toddler on my hands all day. But every so often I would take a deep breath and get on with it, and then I always thought, but this is really nice – why on earth don't we do it more often?'

Some women find that the more they make love, the more they feel like making love, while the longer they abstain, the more that side of themselves seems to shut down and the less they feel like sex. In other women, not feeling like making love is a symptom of depression and lack of positive feelings for themselves as a mother.

'It took months for me to realise that my lack of interest in sex was really a symptom of a postnatal depression. I felt so uninteresting, so ugly, and so low in self-esteem that I didn't understand why anyone would want to make love to me.'

While partners should be sympathetic, understanding and supportive at this time, and most are, there are also some who, not finding sex inside the marriage, look for it elsewhere. If the infidelity is found out, this can lead to a terrible sense of shock and betrayal on the part of the wife, though many marriages survive an infidelity. Fear that their husbands may be driven elsewhere if they don't provide at least a minimum of sex is one reason why many women say they have sex after childbirth: 'It wasn't for me, I could take it or leave it, and would have been happier to leave it. But I couldn't help feeling sorry for him, and I didn't want him to get so desperate he'd start looking elsewhere.'

Perhaps the best solution is for husbands to be actively involved in childcare, getting up in the night, and so on. Then they may also feel too exhausted to want sex.

Going back to work

Making the decision of whether or not to go back to work after having the baby can be an agonising one. Whatever their intentions, some mothers find that they decide in the end not to go back to work. This is most common when the mother's only option is to go back to full-time work, and where the money is not critical.

'I hadn't expected to find motherhood so fulfilling,' says Karen, who was 40 when her first child was born. 'I feel very lucky that I didn't have to go back to my job. This is my full-time job, the most important one there is. It would be crazy for me to be paying someone else to do what really matters while I'm out there pushing pieces of paper around.'

The financial equation can be important. 'I worked out what going back to work was going to bring in after I'd paid for childcare, fares and lunches, and after I'd paid tax. It wasn't worth it,' says one mother who considered going back to teaching. 'I decided to wait until the children were in school.' Other families are not in such a fortunate position. Carol found that working part-time in a clothes shop, after childcare and other expenses she was bringing in £30 a week. Her husband was on a low income and this £30 made all the difference. 'People would say to me, "Why do you do this? It isn't worth it for £30." And I would say, "Of course it's worth it. With that £30 I pay for the week's food."'

Other women work because they cannot risk losing their job and may well find that the opportunities are not there in a few years' time; this is particularly true at a time of high unemployment. 'I knew that the children would become more expensive and that while we could afford for me not to work now, that might not be true in five years' time. I wasn't confident I would get a job once I'd been away for a few years; people would have forgotten who I was.'

In fact women who choose not to work may find that when they try to go back it isn't easy. 'All the women I knew who hadn't had children were in high positions, and now there were all these young people coming in underneath me and at the level that I was. I realised that they didn't want people with my age and experience in these jobs, they wanted bright young things. I realised it was going to be very much more difficult to get back into work than I had originally thought.'

Childcare

Finding adequate child care is also an important part of making the choice. 'At first I found the idea of leaving her with anyone terrifying,' recalls Gillian. 'I found getting

adequate child care a nightmare. I got a list of local authority registered child-minders, but when I went to visit the first
one and found a woman with three other children in a
dreary concrete high-rise estate I just thought, no. In the end
I paid a fortune for a series of nannies; they were all OK, but
none of them stayed for much more than six months.'

Very few companies provide crèches or nurseries, and
local authorities have few day care facilities and these are
mostly filled by single or special needs mothers. Private
nurseries are few and far between and tend to be too expensive for most working mothers. Child-minders can be a
good and inexpensive option if you find one you like.
Nannies can live in if you have space, or can come in for
the day – if you have one child or work part time you may
be able to share a nanny with another mother, thus cutting
costs. Au pairs can work out if you have space and work
part time, but shouldn't be expected to work more than five
hours a day and may be very young and inexperienced with
small children.

Finding suitable child care arrangements is often an on-
going worry for the working mother for many years. What
suited when you have one baby will not suit when you
have two pre-school children, and often child care problems get worse when children start school, because it's
harder to find someone who wants to work only for two or
three hours after school or during school holidays – and
then what do you do when your child is ill? Having both
children and a job usually means that you must have a rea-
sonably understanding relationship with your employer,
that you must be prepared to sacrifice some paid leave for
when your child or child carer is ill, and that your partner
is prepared to make some of these sacrifices too. Otherwise,
the situation may become unworkable.

Giving up work

Older mothers who have had fertility problems are perhaps more likely than others to give up work for the baby. 'They weren't very sympathetic about my taking maternity leave,' says Frances, 'though they accepted I had the right. But they put me under pressure to come back early. I was breast feeding and I didn't want to stop. Then I thought, this is ridiculous. It's taken you six years to have this baby, you'd better make the most of it. So I gave in my notice.'

Not all women have a choice. Although it is against the law, some employers do use pregnancy as a reason to dismiss someone. 'They did it in a very sneaky way, restructuring the whole department, changing the job titles, but basically everything was the same except that I went,' says Yvonne, who got pregnant at 38. 'I didn't go to the industrial tribunal because I don't think I could have proved anything and I did get some freelance work from them which fitted in with the baby and which I wouldn't have got if I'd taken them to court.'

Women who chose their career

For some women, their career is very important and it's clear from the beginning that they will take maternity leave and go back to work, full time or sometimes part time, if this is possible. Increasingly, perhaps because of the recession and the fact that a second income may be vital for the family, women are going back to work sooner.

Maternity leave legislation passed in the 1970s has made it much easier for women to combine a career and family. The legislation means that most women can take up to 29 weeks off work after the birth of the baby and return to the same job they had before. In a few cases this doesn't work; for instance if the woman works part time, under 16 hours a week, or if she is working for a small organisation with fewer than five employees.

Despite this legislation, however, some women feel their career will be affected by having a child. While some organisations are very supportive of working mothers, others – especially some commercial companies – will not promote a woman once she has a family because they believe she may be unreliable, taking time off work to be with sick children, or that she may not stay.

Some women find that they have to work extra hard to convince people that their work has not suffered because they are parents. The kind of work she is doing is also important. 'I had to give up my job as a press officer for a big company because I was expected not just to work nine to five, but to be there in the evening whenever there was a press story, to attend conferences and meetings, and to be available at all times to write a speech or statement. It simply wasn't possible to do this and see my child.'

Some women who decide that career must come first make quite big sacrifices. At 43, with two young children, Judy decided to rent a flat in London. 'I decided in the end that I would stay in a flat in town during the week and go home at the weekends. That way I could dedicate the week to my job and be available all the time, and I could give my weekends up to the children. They were always in bed by the time I got home anyway, so they weren't really missing much. We had an excellent and experienced nanny and I don't think the children have suffered in any way.'

Fiona made the same choice, working more than full time and spending only some weekends with her baby. It worked well till the baby was about nine months old, when he started crying and reaching out for his nanny every time Fiona picked him up. When he was a year old he still wouldn't go to her, so she gave up work and is now at home full time with him and baby number two.

There are other ways around this problem; one older mother and her husband bought a house ten minutes away from the law practice in which she worked. 'It meant I could pop home at lunchtimes for a quick breast feed and to spend half an hour with the children,' she says. 'Sometimes I would come home for an hour or so in the evening to bath them and read a story and then pop back to the office for another stint of work.'

Older women may feel they can't take a few years off when they have a family, because they won't have the time or energy to climb up the ladder again afterwards. Those who do opt to put family first may regret it. Pauline, 38, with one son and then twins, was offered a job with an independent film production company which she turned down. 'The twins were still very little and I wanted to be with them.' Now they are all at school she is looking for work but it isn't available. 'Did I make a mistake? I don't know.'

Sex roles and division of labour

One of the most consistent findings of transition to parenthood studies is that the division of labour becomes more traditional after the birth of the first child. It doesn't seem to matter if the couple used to split tasks 50–50 or if the new mother returns to a full-time job. Inevitably one partner feels put upon; usually it's the mother. One study showed that where families were role reversed and father was at home while mother worked full time, the mother still performed 49 per cent of child care tasks.

'I think it's all right if you've sorted out the roles before-hand – he is Daddy and earns the money and you are Mummy and look after the baby. But we were both doc-tors, both working, and trying to do everything in a not very well-defined way. So we ended up arguing a lot of the time. I would say, "I've had a heavier day than you, so it's your turn to change the nappy." And he would say, "Yes, but I spend more hours in the surgery and I got up twice in the night . . ." We were both so tired we were just trying to put as much as possible onto the other person, and the results were we were always trying to trade things off against the other. But you can't. Does two nappy changes equal one getting up in the night? You just can't do it.'

Part-time working mothers often suffer the worst; they are at home part of the time, and in this time they are expected to do all the things like taking the baby to the doc-tor or health clinic, go for check-ups themselves, do the shopping and washing, clean the house. If the baby is ill it is they who have to take time off to look after him, often working extra hours in lieu so that they are not in trouble at work. Couples find that they have little room for manoeuvre; if one is late they call the other to go home and relieve the child-minder, but this endless juggling often leads to rows.

'You're never in the right place at the right time as a working mother.' Lindsay had her son at the age of 41 and went back to work with an independent production company full time when her son was six months old. She stuck it for six months. 'I found a very experienced and reliable nanny, but once she rang just as I was going into a meeting to say my son's temperature was 103 and should she call the doctor, and did I want to come home. I had to sit through the meeting and I couldn't concentrate on a single word.' Her son always seemed to be ill; in the end the guilt was intolerable.

Cathy went back to work at 45 when her children were 5 and 7. 'The little one started school and I thought, that's it, back to work. It was a disaster. The very first day at my job the school rang to say that the children hadn't been collected. The au pair, who I thought was reliable, had got on a bus going the wrong way and got completely lost. I had to leave and collect them. The very next day, just before I had to take minutes at a big meeting, the school rang to say my seven-year old had fallen over in the school playground and needed stitches in his head. So I had to leave again. I sat with him as his head was stitched and thought, "I have to be here for them. The au pair isn't good enough."'

Positive feelings

Yet, despite all the difficulties, most mothers still speak positively about the experience of older motherhood. Those women who have been mothers before, and have a late child, often in another relationship, make interesting comparisons with how they were as young mothers and older ones. 'I feel I'm a much better parent now than I was then,' says Hilary. 'Then I felt trapped, I wanted to get out and about, I felt restricted. Now I find I can take things slowly, I don't expect to get a lot done, I know this baby will only be small for a very short time and so I'm quite content to take things slowly and just take each day as it comes.'

Some older second time mothers feel that they need less support: 'I knew what I was doing, I suppose, and so I didn't get stressed the way I did with my first child. I also didn't feel the need to get out all the time – I didn't want to go out to playgroups all the time, I didn't want to have other mothers and children round to tea. I thought I could live without that.' Others say their child care approach is more relaxed: 'I don't have such high standards now, I know that it doesn't matter. Sometimes she has a bad day or develops some horrible habit and I just think, she'll grow out of it. With my first child if she didn't eat her carrots my whole day was ruined.'

Research into how older mothers react to motherhood has been carried out by Kate Windridge and Judy Berryman at Leicester University. They studied 346 mothers who had had their babies at 40 or over, 100 of whom were first time mothers. Sixty-three per cent of first time older mothers thought that they would be more tired than they might have felt having one in their twenties, but less than half the second time mothers indicated this, including those who had been mothers in their twenties, too. One-third did mention sleep as a high priority when they had time without their child.

One finding was that babies born to women in their twenties and thirties were more likely to be described as 'difficult' babies than those born to women in their forties. First time older mothers felt that they had greater patience because of their age, and the majority of women with previous children felt that they were more relaxed than with their first borns.

The overwhelming response to motherhood was very positive. These older mothers frequently stated that they were more 'ready' for the demands of a baby and that they didn't miss the curtailment in the social lives. More first time mothers said they would like more time away from their baby and with their partners. Over 90 per cent said that they enjoyed the experience.

Only a tiny percentage (2 per cent) said that it had been a bad experience. However, most reported that the responses of family and friends were of shock, horror and disgust, confirming many older mothers' view that our society is prejudiced against older parents.

Looking ahead

As the children get beyond the baby stage, new difficulties can appear.

'I think one problem for the older mother is that you hit your real mid-life crisis at the same time as motherhood, and this tends to intensify everything. If you are 25 when you have a baby, you can think you'll get into a career when they start school and so on, you have all your life before you. When you have your children, as I did, at 39 and 41, when they start school you're 45. What have you done with your life? Can you stand the strain of motherhood and work? Are you too old to get back into your career? In a few years you're coping with the menopause, with a host of emotional reactions, and you've still got to be a mother meeting the demands of very young children.'

'Having a baby late – and an older husband – meant I had to cope with a lot of problems all at once. I had to cope with finding the right school for my five-year-old child, toddler tantrums, go to the hospital with my husband for investigations into his heart problem, and deal with the heavy bleeding which seemed to be a precursor to the menopause.'

Looking ahead to when children are older, the majority of mothers did not seem to anticipate any particular problems in being in their fifties when their children were teenagers. 'I think that talk about the "generation gap" is rather a lot of nonsense,' says Karen, who was 39 and 41 when her two sons were born; now she is in her fifties. 'When I compare my sons' friends whose parents are younger I don't see any difference in the children's attitudes to us. It's normal for all children to think their parents are old, fuddy-duddy, out of touch. They love to say, "Oh Mum, surely you've heard of x or y?" In fact, I think there's less of a generation gap than there was between my parents' generation and us; there seemed such a gulf between our parents who were young during the war and we who were young during the sixties, and that's not the case now. Today's kids are just as likely to be listening to sixties music as to nineties and we share some of the same heroes; that certainly wasn't true of my parents!'

Older mothers who have teenagers and young babies in the house may find the generation gap has another angle. 'My teenage son wants to play his music, have friends in and be generally noisy, just when the baby's finally settled and I'm in need of peace and quiet. And then there are times when he wants help with his homework and the baby is screaming and needs attention. So it's a complex juggling act. On the other hand, Sam can be wonderfully kind and attentive to the baby and sometimes he's a great help; he'll babysit for a short while or make me a cup of tea when I'm dead on my feet.'

Teenagers with young half-brothers and sisters often oscillate between rapt attention and delight, and disgust and utter boredom, depending on their mood. 'I think the important thing is to divide attention fairly equally, to give the older ones their time and the young ones theirs, and not expect the whole family to revolve around the baby,' says Sarah, with two teenagers from her first marriage and a toddler and baby from her second.

Better late than never?

The overwhelming majority of older mothers do not regret what they've done. 'Most people don't regret being born, and most people don't regret being a mother either,' says one older mother with two young children. 'Once they are there, you love them, and that's the end of it. You sacrifice yourself, you do things you would never believe yourself capable of for them, you would die for them, and you love them with a kind of love that's completely different from anything else you've ever known. On the other hand, if any of us knew what lay ahead, who among us would ever be a mother?'

Further reading

There is a multitude of books available today on pregnancy, childbirth, parenting and also on infertility, miscarriage. This list is a personal one of those books which the author feels may be particularly useful for older mothers. Some of these books may be out of print, but you can always order them from your local library.

Bruno Bettelheim, *A Good Enough Parent*, Thames and Hudson, 1987.

Susan Borg and Judith Laskel, *When Pregnancy Fails – Coping with Miscarriage, Stillbirth, and Infant Death*, Routledge, Kegan Paul, 1982.

Nancy Durrell McKenna, *Birth*, Bloomsbury, 1988.

Deborah Fowler, *A Guide to Adoption: The Other Road to Parenthood*, Optima, 1993.

Judith M Gansburg and Arthur P Mostel, *The Second Nine Months – The Sexual and Emotional Concerns of the New Mother*, Thorsons, 1985.

Jeremy Hamand, *Father over Forty: Becoming an Older Father*, Optima, 1994.

Rachel Holme, *Pregnancy and Diet*, Penguin, 1985.

Maggie Jones, *Infertility*, Piatkus Books, 1991.

Sheila Kitzinger, *Pregnancy and Childbirth*, Penguin, 1986.

Brigid McConville, *Mad to be a Mother: Is there life after birth for women today?* Century, 1987.

Joan Michelson and Sue Gee, *Coming Late to Motherhood*, Thorsons, 1984.

Sylvia P Reuben, *It's Not Too Late for a Baby – For Women and Men over 35*, Prentice-Hall, 1980.

Useful addresses

Association for Postnatal Illness
Mother-to-mother support by telephone for mothers who
are suffering from postnatal depression.
25 Jerdan Place
London SW6 1BE
Tel: 0171-386 0868

British Agencies for Adoption and Fostering (BAAF)
Information on adoption and fostering.
11 Southwark Street
London SE1 1RQ
Tel: 0171-407 8800

British Pregnancy Advisory Service
Counselling and termination of pregnancy, morning-after
contraception, vasectomy, sterilisation and reversals.
Austy Manor
Wootten Wawen
Nr Solihull
West Midlands
B95 6BX
Tel: 01564 793225
(London) 0171-222 0985

[handwritten notes: 1st day of last period / 40 wks / usk 12 / 30·12·98 / Anti-natal apptmt. / 0171 828 2484]

Caesarean Support Group
81 Elizabeth Way
Cambridge CB4 1BQ
Tel: 01223 314211

Family Planning Association
Information on contraception, infertility, sexuality and personal relationships.
27–35 Mortimer Street
London W1N 7RJ
Tel: 0171-636 7866

Gingerbread Association for One Parent Families
35 Wellington Street
London WC2E 7BN
Tel: 0171-240 0953

ISSUE – The National Fertility Association
Counselling and information on infertility.
509 Aldridge Road
Great Barr
Birmingham B44 8NA
Tel: 0121 344 4414

The Maternity Alliance
Information on all aspects of maternity care and rights, including maternity leave and benefits.
15 Britannia Street
London WC1X 9JN
Tel: 0171-837 1265

The Miscarriage Association
Support and information on miscarriage and its after-effects.
c/o Clayton Hospital
Northgate
Wakefield WF1 3JS
Tel: 01924 200799

National Childbirth Trust
A nationwide organisation which runs antenatal classes for women and trains breast-feeding counsellors. Runs post-natal support groups and also has support groups for women who have had Caesarean births or other specific problems.
Alexandra House
Oldham Terrace
Acton
London W3 6NH
Tel: 0181-992 8637

National Council for One Parent Families
255 Kentish Town Road
London NW5 2LX
Tel: 0171-267 1361

Overseas Adoption Helpline
Information on how to adopt from overseas.
34 Upper Street
London N1 OPN
Tel: 0171-226 7666

Stepfamily – National Stepfamily Association
72 Willesden Lane
London NW6 7TA
Tel: 0171-372 0844

The Stillbirth and Neonatal Death Society (SANDS)
28 Portland Place
London W1N 4DE
Tel: 0171-436 7940
Helpline: 0171-436 5881

Support After Termination for Abnormality (SAFTA)
29 Soho Square
London W1V 5DE
Tel: 0171-439 6124

TAMBA
Twins and Multiple Births Association
1 Victoria Place
King's Park
Stirling KF8 3QX
Tel: 01986 72080

Index